Kindly Medicine

Kindly

PHYSIO-MEDICALISM

Medicine

IN AMERICA, 1836–1911

❧ ❧ ❧

JOHN S. HALLER, JR.

❧ ❧

THE KENT STATE UNIVERSITY PRESS

KENT, OHIO, & LONDON, ENGLAND

© 1997 by The Kent State University Press, Kent, Ohio 44242

ALL RIGHTS RESERVED

Library of Congress Catalog Card Number 97-11030

ISBN 0-87338-577-2

Manufactured in the United States of America

02 01 00 99 98 97   5 4 3 2 1

Library of Congress Cataloging-in-Publication Data

Haller, John S.

Kindly medicine : physio-medicalism in America, 1836–1911 /

John S. Haller, Jr.

p.   cm.

Includes bibliographical references and index.

ISBN 0-87338-577-2 (alk. paper) ∞

1. Medicine, Physiomedical—United States—History—19th century.

I. Title.

[DNLM: 1. History of Medicine, 19th Cent.—United States.

2. Philosophy, Medical—history—United States.   WZ 70 AA1 H19k   1997]

RV5.H34   1997

610'.973'09034—dc21

DNLM/DLC

for Library of Congress   97-11030

British Library Cataloging-in-Publication data are available.

For

Jim, Judy, Sue, Mary Ann, Dan, Joe, Sally,

& Bill

Seize upon truth wherever found,
On Christian or on Heathen ground;
Among your friends, among your foes—
The Plant's Divine, where'er it grows.

Masthead,

Physio-Medical Recorder, 1852

CONTENTS

ILLUSTRATIONS

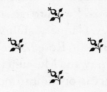

Acknowledgments

Those to whom I am indebted include colleagues Benjamin A. Shepherd, John H. Yopp, Mark Foster, David P. Werlich, David L. Wilson, James Smith Allen, Kay J. Carr, Howard W. Allen, Donald S. Detweiler, John E. Dotson, H. Arnold Barton, David E. Conrad, H. Browning Carrott, John Y. Simon, Julius E. Thompson, Marjorie Morgan, Robbie Lieberman, Rachel Stocking, Edward O'Day, Michael C. Batinski, Tien-Wei Wu, Theodore Weeks, Jerry Lincecum, John Jackson, Glen W. Davidson, Phillip V. Davis, Mary Ellen McElligott, Barbara Mason, Theodore R. Lebang, Carl Getto, Glendon F. Drake, Gilbert Schmidt, James M. Brown, Betty McDowell, Donald W. Wilson, William and Jo Holohan, and Barbara Parker. I am particularly indebted to Alex Berman, professor emeritus of the University of Cincinnati, whose collegial advice and friendship has been sincerely appreciated. Anyone attempting to explore the history of America's botanical movements must, of necessity, begin with his exceptional research. I am also grateful to my wife, Robin, who, as with all of my research, offered inspiration, encouragement, criticism, and substantial assistance, including proofing numerous drafts and indexing the finished manuscript.

Like most authors of historical works, I am especially obligated to the historian-collector-librarians and their professional staffs. Their generosity of time and experienced assistance made possible my understanding of the subject matter. I wish to extend my special gratitude to director/librarian Michael A. Flannery, archivist William C. Black, and staff members Mary Lee Schmidt, Rose Marie Weckenmann, and Betsy Kruthoffer of the Lloyd Library and Museum in Cincinnati, Ohio. Each provided invaluable assistance in opening to me the resources of the Lloyd Library and its wonderful collection on the botanic reformers in American medicine. Without their assistance this book could not have been written. Other librarians to whom I am indebted include Kathy Fahey, Karen Drickamer, James W. Fox, Mary Anne Fox, Kimbra Stout, Andrew Tax, Harry Davis, Iva McRoberts, and Carolyn Synder of the Morris Library of Southern Illinois University, Carbondale; Connie Poole and Jeff Martin from the Southern Illinois University School of Medicine Library; Roger Guard from the University of Cincinnati Medical Library; Martha E. Wright, Pamela Wasmer, and Nancy Eckerman of the Indiana State Library in Indianapolis; and Peter Hirtle and Margaret Kaiser at the National Library of Medicine. Finally, my gratitude would not be complete without noting the fine libraries whose collections I used. These include the Medical Library of Southern Illinois University School of Medicine, Springfield; Denison Library of the University of Colorado Health Sciences Center, Denver; the University of Oregon Medical School Library, Eugene; the University of Utah Library, Salt Lake City; Kent State University Library; Indiana State University Library, Terre Haute; Indiana State Library, Indianapolis; Drake University Library, Des Moines; the University of California at Irvine Medical Sciences Library; Indiana University Library, Bloomington; Johns Hopkins University Library, Baltimore; the Library of Congress; the National Library of Medicine, Bethesda, Maryland; and the Center for Research Libraries, Chicago.

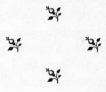

Introduction

Thirteen physio-medical colleges were established between 1836 and 1911—nine prior to 1861, three in the latter decades of the nineteenth century, and one in 1902. By the time Abraham Flexner reported to the Carnegie Foundation in 1910 on the status of medical education in the United States and Canada, only the College of Medicine and Surgery (Physio-Medical) of Chicago, a hybrid descendant of the Physio-Medical Institute of Cincinnati, remained to carry on the reform tradition. The physio-medical system of medical therapeutics, also called sanative medicine, originated with the founding of the Botanico-Medical College and Infirmary in Columbus, Ohio, in 1836. The physios, as they were popularly known, were the direct descendants of Samuel Thomson who began practicing his system of botanic medicine in 1805. Under the leadership of Alva Curtis (1797–1881), a Thomson disciple, the physios emerged as a separate school, teaching and practicing a highbrow formulation of Thomsonian medicine. When the last college closed in 1911, the only surviving element of reform Thomsonism in the United States died with it.

Physio-medicalism was based on principles founded in science, art, and reformation. The scientific principles involved abandoning all mineral drugs, substituting botanical medicines, and denying all chemical or materialistic theories of life. In artistic theory, the physios emphasized the role of the physician in assisting the *life power* or *vital principle* in every patient by using only those measures that were in harmony with the inherent power of the body's vital force. As reformers, the physios demanded the same recognition accorded other schools of medicine: the opportunity to work in army and navy hospitals, asylums, and other public institutions; to receive the same legal rights as any other school of medicine; to have equal representation on all state medical boards; and to obtain exemption from any professional "rulings" that were made in the absence of their representation. Throughout their history, the physios made every effort to characterize regular or allopathic medicine as the mirror image of religious orthodoxy and themselves as righteous and patriotic reformers seeking a more volunteeristic approach to healthcare.[1]

The events and circumstances that brought these practitioners into existence is the context for only a part of this study. Also important is why so few institutions teaching physio-medicalism were chartered, why they experienced such short professional life, and why they all closed by 1911. Certainly part of the explanation is to be found in the competition, rancor, and confusion that reigned between and among the reform partisans of Thomsonism. In this sense, their brief existence is due partly to their own idiosyncracies. A further explanation can be seen in those events that were distancing regular medicine from its earlier rationalistic origins to a grounding in laboratory and clinical science. By midcentury, regular medicine had captured title to science and its new-found status in a century bent on progress.

By contrast, the physio-medicals preferred ideology to the rigors of science and procrastinated when it came to building a curriculum with sound laboratory and clinical experiences for their students. As reluctant participants in the changing medical environment, they found themselves isolated from endowment support, ostracized from scientific and professional associations, suspect before state examining and licensing boards, and viewed increasingly in the public arena as a quaint relic of an earlier age. Belatedly the physios tried to pull the mantle of science over their activities. This proved to be a desperate gamble that ultimately failed. Unable to retain public respect or to finance the changes needed to update their curriculum and facilities, they withdrew from the field—defeated and forgotten.

This study of physio-medicalism is arranged into seven chapters to account for both the institutional development of reformed medicine as well as its theoretical underpinnings. Chapter 1 provides an overview of medical therapeutics and medical education in the opening decades of the nineteenth century. It describes the principal schools of medicine—allopathy, homeopathy, Thomsonism, and eclecticism—and explains the differences that were accepted and practiced among them. Chapter 2 recounts the early defections from Thomsonism and the rise of the independent Thomsonians under the leadership of Alva Curtis. The chapter also traces the development of physio-medicalism, the feud between Alva Curtis and William H. Cook, and Curtis's eventual slide into diploma selling. The focus of chapter 3 is on the history of the first six physio-medical schools and their demise as a result of having adopted the more liberal philosophy of eclecticism and its short-lived advocacy of so-called concentrated medicines. Chapter 4 recounts the development of the two leading physio schools in the second half of the nineteenth century, the Physio-Medical Institute of Cincinnati and the Physio-Medical College of Indiana. Chapter 5 shifts the focus of physio-medicalism away from the institutional history of its colleges and directs attention to the theory of vitalism and the nature of the reform materia medica. Although this chapter could have been inserted earlier in the book, its later placement is intended to simplify the identity of physio teachers and their institutions. Chapter 6 recounts the history of physio-medicalism's national organization, its feuds and fancies, as well as its slow descent into anonymity. Finally, chapter 7 addresses the characteristics of modern medicine as an applied science and the futile efforts of the last several physio colleges to keep abreast of change. It recounts the closing of the last school and assesses physio-medicalism within the botanic movement and in the larger scheme of medical reform.

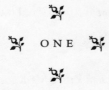

The Medical Landscape

In the opening decades of the nineteenth century, aspiring doctors entered medical practice through a number of different portals. There were those who studied only in the office of a preceptor before entering practice; those whose education consisted of a course of medical lectures without apprenticeship; some who combined apprenticeship or home pupilage in a hospital with a course of lectures at a medical school; those who chose European study, usually following a course of medical lectures in a local medical college; and those who, after some form of self-education, obtained county board approval and began to practice medicine. This mixed character of medical education sparked a debate both within and outside medicine on the essential elements of professional identity that seemed not to resolve itself until the 1870s, when medicine embarked on a course that objectified disease treatment by tying it irrevocably to university-based empirical laboratory science. Until then, nineteenth-century medicine was about differences that were both accepted and practiced among all manner of healers. With the acquisition of new epistemological methods, and with recognition that medical departments must be transformed into more rigorous professional schools modeled on the German ideal, the iconography of American physicians changed. This transformation, however, came as no sudden event but as a series of incidents that started with the spread of democratic medicine and the subsequent rise of French empirical thinking and that eventually signaled a change in traditional medicine and its therapeutic practices.

Democratic Medicine

The democratization of American medicine grew from the same seeds of economic self-sufficiency and high-flown rhetoric that accompanied the speculative commercialism of early nineteenth-century capitalism. Assisted by an applied science that had cast loose from its contemplative moorings, medicine became an instrument of democratic culture, claiming a place that only in time would be justified by actual performance.

One characteristic of this tumultuous new medical democracy was the commercialization of medical education that began with the founding of the College of Medicine of Maryland in 1807. Prior to this time, medical schools were associated with colleges and universities or affiliated in some manner with a medical society. The opening of the Maryland school signaled the start of an indigenous American phenomenon known as the proprietary medical school, separate from any university or parent institution. Organized without collegiate or hospital connections, these schools were little more than for-profit fiefdoms created by local physicians who, in the absence of state boards and examiners, traded diplomas for increased status and income. In most university-affiliated schools, students continued to receive sound medical education in the basic sciences and some level of supervised clinical experience. However, the most that students from proprietary schools could expect from their tickets were lectures supplemented by a few texts, a library collection that often existed in name only, an occasional skeleton or mannequin, and cadavers resurrected under suspicious circumstances. Clinical education, which had been the purpose and intent of apprenticeship, now was eclipsed by didactism and rote repetition of lessons that turned the curricula of these proprietary schools into perfunctory exercises.

As schools proliferated and competition increased in the first half of the century, most medical colleges—including those with university affiliations—chose to attract their share of the student market through a combination of minimal entrance requirements, shortened curricula and terms, reduced matriculation and lecture fees, and lowered graduation expectations. By 1840, twenty-six schools had formed, and another forty-seven would organize over the next forty years. By 1876, sixty-four medical schools were operating in the United States, a number that would climb to 133 by 1890, and to 160 by 1900. No fewer than 308 medical departments formed between 1765 and 1913, plus an additional 118 institutions of highly questionable character.[1]

Until the late 1830s, state medical societies were moderately successful in controlling the legal rights of medical healers through examinations and licenses. But in the new egalitarian environment of post-Jacksonian America, where licensure was equated with elitism, the diminution in the legal power of licensure encouraged the growth of a medical marketplace where phrenologists, occultists, apparatus healers, herbalists, and Indian doctors claimed equal access before the law to practice their profession. By midcentury medical licensure all but disappeared as legislatures dismantled its more restrictive aspects. Anyone with a degree from an unchartered school, or whose education had come entirely by the apprenticeship system, or by some manner of self-proclaimed identity, could set up practice alongside graduates of more conventional schools. All were considered practitioners in the public's eye and before the law. A successful practice rather than an educational pedigree became the true test of a physician's legitimacy.

The legislative response to this new democracy reflected the public's lack of distinction between the competing claims of regulars and various nondescript lay healers. As John Harley Warner explained, "Professional identity was principally based upon practice, not, as it became to a large extent after the late nineteenth century, upon a claim to special knowledge."[2] Above all else, physicians were practitioners in the art of therapeutic intervention. In fact, one could probably discover a greater diversity in practice between geographical regions and among individual physicians than between the various therapeutic systems. In many areas of the country, old-school medicine was held in no higher regard than irregular or sectarian medicine and represented just another school of therapeutic thought. With the waning of apprenticeships (which had long been a tradition in American medical education), the absence of licensing standards, the proliferation of proprietary schools based principally on didactic teaching, and the predisposition of American society to celebrate a volunteer approach to institutional pluralism, there emerged a bifurcated medical education system, both levels of which operated in relative freedom from regulation and restraints. Not surprisingly, medical education became increasingly the target of public derision.

It would be wrong, however, to argue that the art and science of medicine was any worse than before, since many university-based medical schools improved during these years, counteracting the trend toward democratization by emphasizing the importance of basic medical science, by adding sessions before and after the regular term, and by encouraging a continuation of studies in the medical capitals of Europe. During these years, better trained regulars distanced themselves from their less-educated colleagues by identifying with professional societies and gaining control over most city hospitals. Yet, few legal barriers existed to exclude sectarians and lesser-educated regulars from treating willing patients; and physicians could still enter practice without having held an apprenticeship or, for that matter, without ever having had clinical or hospital experience.

Those American physicians who continued to value traditional medical training celebrated the emergence of the Parisian clinical school, which became, in the first half of the nineteenth century, the choice of students seeking a respite from the speculative theories of the day. Empirically oriented and determined to avoid the comfort of prior system builders, this school of thinking—dominated by Philippe Pinel (1745–1826), Jean N. Corvisart des Marets (1755–1821), and Pierre J. G. Cabanis (1757–1808)—held that the bedside was the proper place for instruction of doctors. Eschewing any theory that contradicted facts derived from observation, adherents to the Parisian school of clinical research demanded judgment, strict logic, and a healthy skepticism. The subsequent growth and respectability of empirical philosophy and the objectivity encouraged by the numerical method made possible the identification of specific diseases on the basis of extensive clinical and postmortem examinations. Along with this effort came therapeutic moderation, an emphasis on the healing power of nature, and the overthrow of several traditional therapeutic remedies, including the popular use of bloodletting and reckless dosages of mercury and tartar emetic.[3]

While late eighteenth- and early nineteenth-century America fostered an environment favorable to idiosyncratic practice, by midcentury, as William G. Rothstein has explained, medicine entered a period of transition to a more standardized system of medical practice caused principally by the very multiplicity of medical schools. From fewer than 250 graduates from American medical departments before 1800, to more than 4,000 by 1829, and to 17,000 graduates between 1850 and 1859, medicine took on characteristics that motivated similarly educated doctors to reach a more consensus-driven set of standards. The combination of new schools (including marginal ones), medical and scientific societies and journals, and licensing boards, albeit only honorific, resulted in a set of shared values that ultimately became the basis of physicians' views about themselves and their practice.[4]

With the exception of the Committee on Medical Education, which the American Medical Association appointed in 1848 to prepare annual reports on the general condition of medical education in the United States and abroad, reform mindedness remained in large measure with individuals and a few select schools.[5] The committee (consisting of A.H. Stevens, Amos Twitchell, B.R. Wellford, A. Naudain, R.D. Arnold, and L.P. Bush) reported that the supply of medical doctors exceeded demand. It laid fault for this first on the willingness of private teachers to take on pupils without concern for the students' preliminary education. Secondary responsibility went to the faculty of the medical colleges who, in their "zeal for teaching," admitted too many students lacking in theoretical and practical preparatory instruction. "Were the preliminary qualifications requisite to an admission into private offices and into the medical colleges more enlarged, were the diploma to be purchased only at a mental expenditure corresponding with its value," the committee's report concluded, "not only would the standing of the profession be exalted and its usefulness augmented, but the cause of humanity more truly subserved."[6]

The committee earnestly requested hospitals to open their wards for clinical instruction and to avoid appointing physicians and surgeons on other than strict professional standards. The committee also urged medical schools to build their curricula on practical demonstration and clinical training; insist on a preliminary education for medical students; carefully examine students after attendance at lectures; conduct final examinations of candidates for the diploma "in the presence of some official person . . . who has no pecuniary interest in the institution"; replace the inaugural thesis for the diploma with reports based on personal observations of disease; and maintain accurate records of the number of students and graduates.[7] These recommendations, with modest variations, remained an integral part of the committee's attitude toward medical education through most of the nineteenth century. Over and over again, it drew unkind comparisons between the European system and that of the United States.

Most medical colleges gave little more than lip service to the committee's opinions, knowing that without structural and fiscal reorganization applicable to *all* schools, its recommendations would spell economic disaster for the individual college. No one school could afford to reform unless the rest followed. Moreover, the American Medical Association remained divided over the questions of *who* should study medicine; whether school curricula should be focused on practical medicine or scientific medicine (specialism); what constituted a good general preparation for the study of medicine (i.e., liberal and humanistic studies versus scientific disciplines); the appropriate relationship between the preceptor and the medical college; and the correct relationship between medical colleges and local, state, and national medical organizations. Repeatedly, the association divided on these issues, with men like Martyn Payne of the Medical Department of New York University accusing the educational reform element of attempting to foist an essentially foreign and aristocratic bias on American medical education.[8]

As Kenneth M. Ludmerer has explained, the American Medical Association's actual role in the reform of medical education was more myth than fact. Aside from its published rhetoric, the organization "played no role in either the genesis or implementation of the new ideas of how to teach medicine. Indeed, for most of [the nineteenth] century, the AMA did not even believe in the importance of the scientific subjects, laboratory teaching, or clinical clerkships." Reform, when discussed at all, focused more on the "trappings" than on substantive educational issues.[9]

In this laissez-faire environment where medical colleges jostled one another for credible identities, the relationship between and among schools reflected a curious combination of contentious rivalry, deep-seated jealousy, admiration, and uncontrolled competition. Underlying this rancorous environment was the realization that each school was challenging the other's hegemony by competing for students and patients and using an assortment of claims and counterclaims to vindicate its position.[10]

Allopathy

Foremost among these competing groups were the so-called regulars or *allopaths*. Allopathy was a term first coined by Samuel Christian Hahnemann (1755–1843), the founder of homeopathy, and made popular by his followers in the nineteenth century to distinguish themselves from old-school medicine. It was a term intended to reduce regulars to the same level and legal standing as sectarians, thus denying them any special claim to legitimacy. This suited sectarians just fine, but regulars fought efforts to so stereotype them, viewing the term as intentionally discourteous and relegating them in the public eye to simply another school of medical thinking. Ironically, the term continues in use today among regular medical doctors who seem to have little knowledge of its textual origins.

From the perspective of modern (scientific) medicine or, at least until the full impact of the Paris clinical school on medical education, early nineteenth century allopathy was little different from other schools of medicine since, like them, it was grounded in speculative rationalism. "Prior to the placing of medicine on a scientific basis," wrote educator Abraham Flexner, author of *Medical Education in the United States and Canada* (1910), "Sectarianism was . . . inevitable. Every one started with some sort of preconceived notion; and from a logical point of view, one preconception is as good as another. Allopathy was just as sectarian as homeopathy." From Flexner's perspective, what regulars viewed as correct medicine represented little more than a relic of an extinct science, a dead husk that had taken the form of dogma.[11]

The term *allopathy* (derived from the Greek word *allos,* or different, and *pathos,* meaning disease) denoted the method of curing disease by means of remedies that were believed to act contrary to the nature of the disease. This method was based on the proposition that *first,* no two diseases could coexist in the body at the same time; and *second,* that diseases were best cured by establishing artificially morbid conditions of a different character that would substitute for the disease itself. Affected tissues or organs were to be treated by medicinal agents that, if applied to a healthy organism, would produce unhealthy effects. By substituting an artificial diseased action for the disease itself, the allopath could extinguish the original disease and then treat the artificial diseased action as a temporary condition. Implied in this regimen was an important correlation between professional identity and active therapeutic intervention. The integrity of the allopath's healing regimen and the respect due his social standing depended ultimately on his ability to energetically intervene in nature.

The ratiocinations used by regulars to explain their choice of regimens were exemplary of the problems inherent in both the quest for a science of medicine and in allopathy's solipsistic view of disease. In the early nineteenth century, old-schoolers had resorted to heroic bleeding, only to leave off treatment in later decades believing that environmental conditions in America (and presumably Europe as well) had changed, thereby affecting the ability of the human constitution to tolerate excessive depletion. The justification for bleeding had not changed; rather the human constitution had modified, thus necessitating a milder form of treatment.[12] The "old fogy system" of regular medicine would have collapsed decades earlier, argued its critics, had it not incorporated elements of reform into its theory and practice. Indeed, allopathy's fortuitous acquisition of science had so modified "old physic" that it was hardly recognizable in its new clothes.[13]

Allopaths were also criticized for having attached so much emphasis to their materia medica that they seldom recognized the natural operations of the organism, choosing instead to attribute any benefits to their use of drugs and other measures. Thus originated the adage *post hoc, propter hoc*, meaning a patient gets well after taking a medicine, and therefore in consequence of it. Critics accused regulars of opposing all efforts to improve medicine until "they could no longer resist the popular clamor." Only then did they respond by smuggling improvements into their ranks "without giving proper credit to the discoverer." Such, critics argued, had been the circumstances regarding the discovery of the circulation of the blood, the use of Peruvian bark, vaccination, and similar innovations.[14]

Homeopathy

Competing with allopathy was Hahnemann's school of *homeopathy* whose doctrine of *similia similibus curantur*, meaning like cures like, was based on the belief that the curative power of medicines stemmed from their ability to induce in healthy persons symptoms analogous to the diseases for which they were administered. In theory, this meant that doctors should employ purgative medicines in cases of diarrhea, emetic remedies for vomiting, and opium and astringents for costiveness. Hahnemann added to this concept the idea of prescribing minute amounts of medicine, thereby emphasizing its dynamic and spirit-like force rather than its toxic impact. Both he and his followers, many of them graduates of leading European universities, subscribed to the vitalistic approach to medicine, believing that a spirit-like force was present in every organism and that sickness was a morbific agency inimical to life but susceptible to the dynamic impact of highly attenuated medicines. For Hahnemann and his brand of medical reformers, an understanding of vital force was an essential step in the cure of disease since it guided the observant physician to select the proper medicinal agents. Above all else, practitioners of homeopathy relied heavily on observation and experience in the selection of medicines, believing that correct remedies were based on the totality of a person's symptoms. While the allopath admitted that vital force was *sometimes* the cause of disease, Hahnemann went further. Only an "abnormally modified vital force can excite morbid sensations in the organism, and determine the abnormal functional activity which we call disease."[15]

The propositions that defined the system of homeopathy included the following: Disease is purely dynamical (i.e., due to a change in the spiritual nature of man); disease is known only by its symptoms, and therefore the study of pathologies is useless; disease can never be cured by antipathic or allopathic treatment; disease can be cured only by exciting a disease similar to the one the patient suffers; all direct treatment of local disease is wrong; the power of medicine can be ascertained by "provings" on healthy persons; only single remedies should be given at any one time; the effect of a single dose of medicine may last upwards of 100 days; the dose of medicine must be small; a medicine's effectiveness is due to a dynamical or spiritual power conferred on it by shaking or rubbing; it is not always necessary for medicines to be swallowed; smelling is sometimes sufficient; and most diseases are caused by psora, or the itch.[16]

The American homeopaths, beginning with Hans Burch Gram (1788–1840), who began his practice in Boston in 1825 and spread Hahnemann's ideas through the Northeast; Henry Detwiller, a Swiss physician who established the North American Academy of Homeopathic Medicine in Allentown, Pennsylvania, in 1835; Constantine Hering

(1800–1880), known as the father of American homeopathy, who organized the Homeopathic Medical College of Pennsylvania (Philadelphia)
in 1848; and David S. Smith, who organized the Hahnemann Medical
College of Chicago in 1860 and spread the doctrines into the South and
West, offered strong competition to allopathic medicine. Most of the
sect's early converts came from regular practice (i.e., John F. Gray and
Abraham D. Wilson, both students of David Hosack, professor of theory
and practice of physic at the College of Physicians and Surgeons of New
York), a fact especially irritating to regulars and leading eventually
to many bitter feuds. Not only did the homeopaths establish medical
schools and hospitals and produce a plethora of journals and medical
texts, they also received support from the professional and intellectual
elite, making them a strong force to contend with. The fact that homeopaths prospered financially and socially without bleeding or puking
their patients only made their presence that much more of a nuisance to
regulars. By prescribing smaller doses of drugs, opposing polypharmacy,
and relying on the healing power of nature, they offered a more appealing alternative to patients who had wearied of orthodoxy's more drastic
regimens.[17]

Critics called homeopathy a system of "smoke and mirrors," accusing
its practitioners of using the spirit-like powers of bedbugs, spiders, and
other unusual substances in the treatment of disease and of triturating
their medicines upwards of 200 and 300 times their weight in milk sugar
or lactose. That a grain of anthracite coal mixed with twenty or thirty
times its weight in lactose and administered in minuscule amounts could
cure dropsy, skin diseases, sleeplessness, night sweats, fever, dry mouth,
coated tongue, loss of appetite, urinary affections, and diseases of the
genital organs tested the full measure of human credulity.[18]

Despite the efforts of the American Medical Association to use
the consultation clause in its code of ethics to exclude homeopaths as
colleagues in patient consultations, and despite the restriction of homeopaths from many tax-supported hospitals and from army appointments,
homeopathy represented the most respected sect in the nineteenth century. Marks of its success were the opening of medical colleges, including
some with university affiliation; changes in therapeutic practices that
brought allopathy and homeopathy closer together; and the establishment of composite boards to examine applicants for medical licensure.
States with the largest numbers of homeopathic physicians included

New York, Pennsylvania, Ohio, Michigan, Massachusetts, Wisconsin, and Indiana. In 1873, regulars represented 78 percent of the total number of practicing doctors in the United States, followed by homeopaths with 5.9 percent, eclectics with 5.7 percent, and the remainder, nearly 10 percent, consisting of physio-medicals, hydropaths, and various undefined types.[19]

The Botanics

Botanic medicines became the basis for yet another group of practitioners, the majority of whom remained outside any formalized school or party. Based on the premise that God provided every region of the world with its own medicines, early explorers and colonists presumed that a careful cataloging of a region's botanicals and the identification of herbs, barks, and roots used by native peoples would measurably add to the armamentarium of medical knowledge. Herbal medicines became an important part of the age of discovery and exploration with such substances as guaiacum, sarsaparilla, balsam of Peru, cascara sagrada, cocaine, curare, capsicum, arrowroot, cocillana, jalap, and tobacco introduced as new therapeutic substances. Even the English Crown encouraged this activity by ordering colonies to cultivate gardens of natural products to determine their medical (and commercial) use. Before long, American settlers were using sassafras for skin diseases, gout, rheumatism, and syphilis; snakeroot as a tonic, diuretic, diaphoretic, and stimulant in typhoid and digestive disorders; dittany as a purge for worms; jimsonweed as a sedative and antispasmodic; and wild cherry bark as a specific in wounds and sores. Given the high cost of imported chemical and galenical preparations, Americans learned the efficacy of substituting less expensive native botanicals.[20]

The fact that regular doctors, or those trained by more orthodox methods, had come to rely on a native plant materia medica in the early days of the colonies and during the subsequent nation-building years of the young republic speaks to the importance and broad acceptance given to newly discovered plant species. Exemplary of this, John Bartram (1699–1777), a self-educated botanist, established a botanical garden in Philadelphia around 1730, and his cousin, Humphrey Marshall (1722–1801), authored *Arbustrum Americanum, The American Grove*

(1785), a catalog on the Linnaean plan of American trees and shrubs. Other notable efforts included those by physicians Thomas Cadwalader (1708–79), John Redman (1772–1808), and John Morgan (1735–89) who kept "physic gardens" for both teaching purposes and for sources of medicines; Congregational preacher, botanist, and pioneer Manasseh Cutler (1742–1823) of Massachusetts who published *Vegetable Productions, Botanically Arranged* in the proceedings of the Philosophical Society of Philadelphia in 1785; physician-naturalist Benjamin Smith Barton (1766–1815) who prepared the first printed collection of the American materia medica in 1798; and noted physician and political leader Benjamin Rush (1745–1813) who urged the cultivation of botanical gardens by the medical schools of Boston and New York. Indeed, the University of Pennsylvania, Jefferson Medical College, and the Philadelphia College of Pharmacy were all interested in botany as it pertained to the materia medica.[21] As one industrial pharmacist noted, the American materia medica was the work of "the intensely religious, the professionally dogmatic, and the hopefully scientific, as well as the ever-present commercially ambitious, all seeking alike the secrets that reposed in the natural products of the new world."[22]

Outside the boundaries of orthodox medicine, botanic medicines had also become the property of any number of lay-healers—midwives, oculists, apothecaries, bonesetters, surgeon-dentists, Indian doctors, many less formally educated doctors who were self-taught or learned by apprenticeship, itinerant salesmen and preachers, and perhaps most importantly, parents and family friends. Americans, many of whom were versed in domestic medicine and were familiar with European works on the subject, sought substances that possessed qualities similar to those recommended in Cotton Mather's *The Angel of Bethesda* (1722); the many editions of Nicholas Culpeper's *Pharmacopoeia Londinensis* (1649); and Johann David Schoepf's *Materia Medica Americana* (1787).

Not surprisingly, those botanicals with the most appeal also had the greatest aromatic, emetic, cathartic, or energetic quality. Thus sassafras, serpentaria, senega, podophyllum, spigelia, ipecac, cinchona, jalap, hydrastis, and sanguinaria were immediately popular. Given the accepted heroics in therapy that dominated medical practice in the late eighteenth and early nineteenth centuries, it was not at all unusual that the heroic tradition extended as well to the plant materia medica. The advocates of these new medicines took special note of their energetic and disagreeable qualities as somehow proof of their healing effects. The reputed strength of botanicals paralleled the popularity of energetic European drugs and patent medicines—both mineral and vegetable. William P. C. Barton's *Vegetable Materia Medica of the United States* (1818–25) breathed every bit of the spirit of European old-school medicine in which diseases required an energetic if not harsh form of medication to be effective.[23]

Botanicals constituted most of domestic and folk medicine, varying only by region, drug availability, cost, and patient preference. To speak, however, of a botanic *movement* or a standardized system of botanic practice before Samuel Thomson, Alva Curtis, or Wooster Beach (the founders of Thomsonism, physio-medicalism, and eclecticism, respectively) would be a misnomer, for there were only botanic healers, each practicing a very idiosyncratic form of medicine. Many botanic healers had remarkable careers but, for the most part, lived in rural areas and were known only by the families in their region. Similarities that existed across the rural landscape were tenuous at best, subject to the common ownership of a few domestic medicine texts, the spread of popularized remedies, the strength of the oral tradition, the reputation of a particular healer, and the connectivity of roads and water routes. In the absence of medical schools, societies, or journals that in later decades did much to standardize botanical practice, information regarding new botanicals went unnoticed except as happenstance made spread of that knowledge possible.

Thomsonians

Thomsonism had its origins in the observations, experiences, discoveries, and declarations of Samuel Thomson (1769–1843) of Alstead, New Hampshire, who in 1805 founded a system of botanic therapeutics that spread through the Northeast, South, and Middle West with a fervor that paralleled the growth and popularity of religious sectarianism in the early nineteenth century. Little in Thomson's medicine bag was new. Except for the substitution of botanic medicines for mineral-based drugs and an assertion of the inherent power of the body's vital force, the principles of his medical system were surprisingly similar to regular medicine in both philosophy and effect. Nevertheless, his followers credited him with starting "one of the grandest reforms that has ever yet claimed the attention of any people."[24]

As a youth, Thomson had developed a curiosity regarding herbs and spent time accompanying a local herb doctor named Benton on her collecting trips. Soon he became acquainted with the names and uses of various roots and herbs and began to chew plants to learn their taste and their effect on the body. One of his favorites was lobelia (*Lobelia inflata*), which he later called his emetic herb and which, as a child, he sometimes convinced playmates to chew "merely by way of sport, to see them vomit."[25] Lobelia, found in most areas of the United States, had been given the name *Indian tobacco* by the pioneers. Morris Mattson, in *The American Vegetable Practice* (1841) attributed the first use of the herb as a medicine to the Penobscot Indians of New England who reputedly used it for gastritis, asthma, palpitations of the heart, strangury, and nervous affections.[26]

Young Thomson became a local expert on plants and soon was called upon by neighbors to treat their infirmities. At the age of sixteen, he was to have been apprenticed to a root doctor named Fuller, but lacking funds and required by his family to work their farm, he resigned himself to a less formal apprenticeship from two local root doctors and a doctor of mixed (regular and herbal) practice who lived on the Thomson farm.

Thomson married in 1790 and relied on both regulars and root doctors as well as on his own wits to care for his family. Eventually, he concluded that his own herbs were more reliable than anything that regulars could provide. By 1796 he was turning with increasing frequency to a combination of lobelia and steam cure for the treatment of canker-rash (scarlet fever), measles, and various other diseases. By this time his reputation had spread, and he became convinced that he possessed a gift for healing. In 1805, he gave up farming to practice full time as an herb doctor, serving southern New Hampshire, Maine, and northeastern Massachusetts. A year later he opened an infirmary in Boston and, in 1808, took a blacksmith's helper into his practice as an apprentice. By 1810, Thomson had begun manufacturing his special remedies and, three years later, succeeded in obtaining a patent for his healing technique.[27]

The medical theories of Thomson were not too dissimilar from Galen's humoral pathology. Thomson accepted the basic four elements of earth, air, fire, and water (with their qualities of wet, dry, hot, and cold), and he attributed disease to the lessening of heat due to an imbalance of the four humors in the living organism.[28] The object of his therapeutic

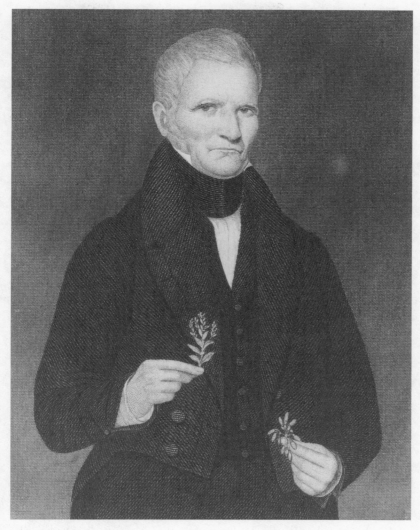

Samuel Thomson (1769–1843) with his lobelia plant. Courtesy of the New York Academy of Medicine.

regimen was to restore the digestive powers thereby increasing the level of heat on which life depended. He condemned bleeding, tartar emetic, and calomel—the three principal weapons of regular practice—as failing to support the body in its cold state of disease.[29]

Thomson's alternative to regular medicine consisted of lobelia ("puke-weed"), hot botanicals such as red pepper, restoratives, and steam therapy. Like allopathy, his system involved considerable unpleasant-ness for the patient since it consisted of regulating the body's secretions through a combination of purging, sweating, and puking. Nevertheless, he touted the method as safe because it used natural herbs rather than harsh minerals. On balance, however, the premises on which allopathy and Thomsonism operated were roughly the same. Both proceeded from a belief that the art of healing lay in modifying the body's secretions. Medical judgment derived from the metaphor of the body as an inte-grated whole and the need for medical intervention to repair any sec-retory imbalances.[30]

Thomson's patented method of cure consisted of a steam bath to add heat to the body, followed by specific vegetable preparations intended to restore the system to its natural health. Steaming involved placing an undressed patient (wrapped in blankets) on a chair; under the chair an operator placed a pan in which red-hot stones were immersed to create steam.[31] Following the steam treatment, Thomson prepared a six-step herbal procedure using emetics, purgatives, enemas, and renewed sweat-ing. He began the process with lobelia in combination with red pepper and brandy to create natural heat, cleanse the stomach, and promote perspiration. After another steam bath, he then prescribed red peppers, ginger, or black pepper to increase heat and continue perspiration. This was followed by a choice of bayberry, the root of white pond lily, the inner bark of hemlock, the root of marsh rosemary, the leaves of witch hazel, the leaves of red raspberry, or squaw weed to "scour the stom-ach and bowels." The next step consisted of a choice of bitters plants (balmony, bitterroot, poplar bark, barberry, or root of goldenseal) to correct the bile and restore the patient's digestion. He then used tonic plants (peach meats or cherry stones) prepared in a mixture of sugar and brandy to strengthen the stomach and bowels. Finally, Thomson pre-scribed his popular Rheumatic Drops (combination of wines or brandy, gum myrrh, and cayenne pepper) to remove pain and restore the body's natural heat. Although Thomson's complete materia medica consisted of seventy different plants, the mainstays of his patented system were lo-belia powder, bayberry root bark in powder, cayenne pepper, ginger, poplar bark, and Rheumatic Drops.[32]

Thomsonism began as a protest against the destructive practice of bloodletting and the harmful use of calomel, tartar emetic, arsenic, and other harsh mineral drugs that had become an essential part of the armamentarium of medical orthodoxy. It was one of a number of reform efforts that emerged following the clamor of an increasingly critical public searching for less drastic remedies in the treatment of disease. But it also attached itself to any number of political and social reforms of the day, including hydropathy, phrenology, mesmerism, grahamism (after Sylvester Graham who popularized the use of graham or whole wheat flour), and Jacksonianism. In hundreds of communities, bands of Thomsonians combined with other reform advocates and carried on vigorous campaigns to enlighten the public to the dangers of old-school medicine and other forms of monopoly and elitism. Even regulars from old-school ranks such as Benjamin Waterhouse (1754–1846) of Harvard, a combative and ardent Jeffersonian, gave public testimony to the merits of Thomson's views and advocated an honest investigation of his claims. Additional support came from physician William Tully (1785–1859) of Yale; physician and naturalist Benjamin Smith Barton of Philadelphia; and abolitionist, grahamite, and temperance advocate William Lloyd Garrison (1805–79).[33]

The particular strength of Thomson's popularity lay in his democratic appeal that offered to all who were willing to pay twenty dollars for rights to his 1813 patent (renewed in 1823 and again in 1837) the opportunity to cure themselves of sickness and disease without dependence on the pretensions of a learned profession. Here was a calling open to men and women alike, a system of self-help that allowed families to support their health needs via a patented process of therapeutic measures. Throughout the heyday of Thomson's leadership, the movement opposed the establishment of medical schools and medical societies—both of which implied the need for a professional medical class. Instead, Thomson (known affectionately as "Old Sammy") substituted a system of medicine fully contained within the do-it-yourself philosophy of the common man. Together with sons Samuel, Cyrus, and John, he carried the message of his botanic cures through New England, western New York, and into Ohio and the Midwest, while disciples and agents, such as clergyman William Fonerden, brought the steam and puke gospel into the South.[34]

Most regulars condemned Thomson as an "ignorant farmer," no different from the numerous root and herb doctors and other empirics who plied their trade across the American countryside in the late eighteenth and early nineteenth centuries. But the marketing success of Thomson's patented system far exceeded what any critics had expected from his "unlettered" background. The principles he advocated in the *New Guide to Health* (1822), and especially the idea of nonpoisonous medication, appealed to a broad spectrum of American society. Indeed, Thomson's patented system offered a nonthreatening alternative to the regulars' reliance on depletive drugs and practices in the treatment of fevers, colic, dysentery, rheumatism, and many other illnesses where sweating was the recognized regimen of choice. By 1849, his book had gone through twenty-six editions.[35]

Agents of Thomson spread his botanic message throughout New England and New York, moving south into Georgia and west into Ohio, Indiana, and Illinois, selling rights to family practice. The *Thomsonian Recorder* listed 167 authorized agents in 1833, and in Ohio alone, it has been estimated that Thomson's herbal medicines were used by almost half the population.[36]

The Eclectics

Another group of botanics to emerge in the 1820s were the eclectics. Known also as the *American School of Medicine*, they were fond of establishing their intellectual origins among pre-Christian healers who chose to select from competing medical opinions those ideas and regimens that had proven most successful. Not until the first century A.D. did these efforts coalesce into the *Episynthetic* school, with Claudius Agathinus of Sparta as the father of this new group. Medical eclecticism emerged again in the seventeenth century with the so-called *eclectic conciliators* who soon disappeared for lack of a unifying theory. Rising once again in France in the early nineteenth century, it represented, according to historian Erwin H. Ackerknecht, "the fourth and last episode in the supremacy of Paris medicine." French medical eclecticism was connected with the philosophical views of Victor Cousin (1792–1867) and combined both skepticism and political liberalism. Medical exponents of this philosophy included G. B. A. Coutanceau, René-Théophile-Hyacinthe Laennec (1781–1826), Louis de Rochefort Desbois, Jean Baptiste Bouillaud (1796–1881), Jules-René Guérin, Gabriel Andral (1797–1876), Armand Trousseau (1801–67), François Magendie (1783–1855), and Pierre Adolphe Piorry (1794–1879) who worked at the Pitié, Salpêtrière,

Charité, and Hotêl Dieu hospitals. There, they employed the numerical method of Pierre Charles Alexandre Louis (1787–1872), emphasized the powers of clinical observation and experimentation, and practiced the technique of auscultation.[37]

In the United States, eclecticism was espoused by Wooster Beach (1794–1868), Ichabod G. Jones (d. 1857), John King (1813–93), and John M. Scudder (1829–94) who, beginning in the 1820s and 1830s, saw their reform movement as an alternative to allopathic practice. They also saw themselves as wholly separate from the steam and puke followers of Thomson. Ostensibly, these American reformers gave deference to French eclecticism, the eclectic conciliators, and earlier groups. In practice, however, the Americans were noticeably different from their intellectual forebears in that, while theoretically open to new ideas and methods, they seemed more intent on eschewing foreign influences for a more nativistic blend of domestic medicine and education.[38]

Wooster Beach, the father of American eclecticism, broke from the traditional practices of earlier botanics to utilize what, for the period, was a gentler materia medica. In his *American Practice of Medicine* (1833), Beach, a graduate of the medical department of the University of New York, showed himself conversant with the botanical literature of the past, including Benjamin Smith Barton's *Collections for an Essay Towards a Materia Medica of the United States* (1798); Constantine Samuel Rafinesque's *Medical Flora: Or, Manual of the Medical Botany of the United States of North America* (1828–30); Johann David Schoepf's *Materia Medica Americana* (1787); the writings of Robley Dunglison (1798–1869) and William Tully (1785–1859); as well as the United States pharmacopoeias of 1820 and 1830. Having adopted the motto of "vires vitales sustinete" or, the vital forces of a patient must be sustained, he moved unhesitatingly to replace the more powerful depletive remedies—both mineral and botanical—with those that were less energetic.

In his efforts to detect the errors of modern practice, Beach began privately instructing students at his New York City home in 1825 and later opened a clinical school known as the United States Infirmary in 1827. In 1829, he enlarged the school, calling it the Reformed Medical Academy; a year later, it bore the name Reformed Medical College of the City of New York.

From this original college sprang the medical descendants of eclecticism, including the medical department of Worthington College in the aspiring village of Worthington, Ohio, a neighbor of Columbus and a hopeful contender for the new capital of Ohio. In 1830, the medical college at Worthington became the first chartered, degree-granting school in the United States dedicated to botanic medicine. Following several defections within its faculty, the machinations of allopathic enemies, and a notorious "resurrection riot" in 1839, the school closed and moved to Cincinnati in the winter of 1842–43 where it reorganized as the Reformed Medical School of Cincinnati and on March 10, 1845, incorporated as the Eclectic Medical Institute. Known affectionately as "EMI," the college became the bastion of reform thinking in the nineteenth and early twentieth centuries, producing the largest number of graduates from eclectic-based medical schools and making the most significant contributions to eclectic theory and practice.

Contemporary critics were fond of calling eclecticism the school of "non-committalism," since it rejected all principles and, instead, celebrated individual choice in the selection of remedies and practices. By acknowledging no external authority and viewing each individual as an authority unto his own, the eclectics could hold no person responsible. In point of fact, however, the eclectics, at least in theory, attempted to break from the dogmatic views of old-school medicine and, like many regular physicians in the 1830s, were enamored by the empirical and diagnostic breakthroughs of the Paris clinical school.[39]

The eclectics were as much opposed to the sweating, vomiting, and heroic regimens of the early botanics as they were to the bleeding, blistering, and mercurial purging and salivating regimens of the regulars. Operating on a parallel but less heroic road to wellness, the eclectics introduced and marketed so-called concentrated medicines, including the resin of podophyllum as a substitute for calomel; used counterirritants to relieve affections; devised a compound tar plaster to replace old-school applications of croton oil, cantharides, and tarter emetic; and used compound tincture of sanguinaria and compound lobelia powder for emesis.[40]

John King, the developer of concentrated medicines and author of *The American Eclectic Dispensatory* (1859), did much to simplify and explain the eclectic materia medica. When, in the mid-1850s, the therapeutic value of concentrated medicines came under criticism because of over-zealous manufacturers and outright adulterations (John King himself denounced the mercenary aspects of his original discovery), eclecticism faced the prospect of being undermined internally by its own medicines. Indeed, this sorry state led many eclectics to abandon the cause. Symptomatic of this malaise, numerous eclectic schools closed, and even the National Eclectic Medical Association, founded in 1848, suspended activities.[41]

Under the leadership of John M. Scudder, the eclectics rebounded by embracing the theory and practice of specific medication. This new doctrine, as elaborated by Scudder in his *Specific Medication and Specific Medicines* (1870) and *Specific Diagnosis* (1874), theorized that a fixed relationship existed between drug force and disease expression. In other words, disease "should not be treated by routine methods, according to disease names, but . . . should be specifically adapted to the particular symptom-complex under observation."[42] This meant specific medication for specific conditions, direct medication for definite states as individually indicated, or special drugs meeting special conditions of disease.[43]

Scudder turned to botanic pharmacist John Uri Lloyd to manufacture his preparations of specific medication. These were simple tinctures made by percolation and based on the motto "vires vitales sustinete." Scudder was sometimes likened to a "pseudo-homeopath" in that his specific doses were small and intended for therapeutic action and not physiological shock. He continued to draw from the botanical medicines of Schoepf, Barton, Thomson, and Beach, but by inaugurating a series of clinical therapeutic investigations that were more systematic than anything previously attempted, he was able to further refine drug applicability while abandoning many less valuable agents, including unnecessary sugar and glycerin and other substances that had been added to medicines.[44]

The eclectics had an affinity to homeopathy that never quite went away, perhaps because all so-called irregulars found common cause in facing the power of old-school medicine. Partly, too, it was due to the strength of homeopathy among many wealthy and cultured Americans who showed an appreciation for the homeopath's microdoses of substances in place of the "sledgehammer" doses then in vogue. True, the homeopath's theory of dynamization was incomprehensible to most eclectics; yet, in general, the eclectics were enamored with homeopathy's minimalist approach and saw excessive doses of innocuous drugs as retarding the body's natural affinity to self-repair.[45]

Over the course of the nineteenth century, some two dozen eclectic schools organized to challenge the errors and extravagances of old-school medicine and to offer a simpler system of botanic medication.

Most of the early eclectic schools closed as a result of the poor publicity attending their concentrated medicines. Others that opened in the second half of the nineteenth century fell slowly by the wayside as regular schools embarked on a course leading to more rigorous academic medicine. By 1905, the approved list of eclectic medical colleges as determined by the National Eclectic Medical Association, organized in 1848, consisted of American Medical College of St. Louis, Missouri; Bennett College of Eclectic Medicine and Surgery of Chicago, Illinois; California Medical College located in San Francisco, California; Eclectic Medical College of the City of New York; the Eclectic Medical Institute of Cincinnati; Georgia College of Eclectic Medicine and Surgery in Atlanta; and Lincoln Medical College in Lincoln, Nebraska.[46]

In the decade that followed, all but one of these schools closed outright or merged with university-based medical colleges. The remaining eclectic college in Cincinnati struggled against impossible odds. Unable to work out a merger with the University of Cincinnati, it failed also to arrange suitable clerkships for its students at the Cincinnati General Hospital. Under pressure from its own graduates who objected to being denied internship and residency opportunities in class "A" hospitals, the school's board of trustees reluctantly closed admission to new students in 1936 and shut its doors for good in 1939.

Angles of Vision

Henry I. Bowditch (1808–92), professor of clinical medicine at Harvard Medical School and president of the American Medical Association, represented a minority among the leaders in American medicine who felt that regular physicians ought to have more humility regarding their claims to orthodox practice; similarly, he rejected the association's dictum not to confer with sectarian practitioners. In counseling his colleagues, he instead urged greater sympathy and understanding. "You have been so accustomed to look down upon these sects," he observed, "that you forget that they have schools where all branches of medicine are taught quite as well as in many of the smaller schools of the country, and vastly better than they were taught fifty years ago in the highest colleges." By opening rather than closing discussion between and among the fraternity of regulars and sectarians, he hoped medicine would eventually evolve to the point of having no distinctive marks to separate them, and that "all will become merged again . . . always imperfect, yet always improving."[47]

In comments written for the *Proceedings* of the Philadelphia County Medical Society in 1899, Edward Jackson, M.D., professor of the diseases of the eye in the Philadelphia Polyclinic, questioned whether allopathy had not overstepped the bounds of ethics in its insistence on the correctness of its ideas. The domain of medicine offered sufficient room for honest differences of opinion. While it was important to encourage professional harmony and cooperation, these had to be balanced with the freedom of individual opinion. He noted that the code of ethics read: "No one can be considered a regular practitioner or fit associate in consultation, whose practice is based on an exclusive dogma to the rejection of the accumulated experience of the profession and of the aids actually furnished by anatomy, physiology, pathology, and organic chemistry." Too many of his allopathic colleagues preferred a narrow interpretation of the term *regular* until it no longer conveyed its proper meaning, namely, that "the person to whom it is applied has had a respectable medical education." Jackson argued that simply belonging to a certain school or sect that differed from allopathy in certain dogmas or doctrines should not be the basis of defining the term regular. Graduates of the Hahnemann Medical College of Philadelphia were no less qualified to practice medicine; a review of their courses and texts indicated that students in the college received no less an education. Of the textbooks used in their studies, two-thirds were written by authors unquestionably orthodox, and the remaining third were from equally creditable authorities. "The medical profession can never afford either to prescribe or proscribe opinions for its members," reminded Jackson. "Whenever you divide medical practitioners upon a line of dogma, whether that line be to include the believers in a certain doctrine or to exclude them, you introduce, with all its evils, sectarianism in medicine." For this reason he believed the American Medical Association had the obligation to bind the profession into a harmonious whole, but not by "false interpretations and failure to comprehend [a] catholic spirit."[48]

The views of Bowditch and Jackson notwithstanding, intolerance, jealousy, and rivalry seemed to reign between and among the various sects, including allopathy. Homeopaths refused to recognize eclectics, and allopaths turned up their noses on all, regardless of their contributions.

Each seemed content to identify with its own and none other. One sectarian observed in a moment of reflection that "there is incompetency enough in any and all schools of medicine and one would suppose that each would have enough to see after to rid itself of the incompetents in its own ranks. . . . Let all strive for the establishment of a science of medicine. In doing this there will be less time for calling others ugly names." His comments, however nobly intended, fell on deaf ears.[49]

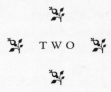

TWO

Thomson's Progeny

Following a decade of authoritarian leadership, Thomson's followers began to establish infirmaries (which Thomson suspected as the beginnings of another medical monopoly) and to advocate formal education in addition to patient practice as essential components of botanic reform.[1] These same individuals expanded Thomson's materia medica to include other potential remedies, most of which the founder vigorously opposed. These deviations from the patented system of herbal medicine resulted in a schism in 1838 marked by the waning of Thomson's personal influence and the emergence of new leadership.[2]

The criticism leveled at Thomson was that he limited the practice of his therapeutic system only to those who had purchased rights to his patent. He and his closest disciples opposed the establishment of medical colleges, insisting that medical education had been transformed into the private reserve of educational elitists. Instead, Thomson established Friendly Botanical Societies to share information and cures and thereby bridge differences in individual practice and experience. According to botanic reformer E. Anthony, writing in 1886, those who cast their lot with Thomson and followed his example turned against formal medical

education and the organization of medical colleges. Nevertheless, it became "plainly evident that uneducated men could not any longer compete with those who possessed even a meager collegiate education."
Given the predicament Thomson had forced on the botanics, and believing that his narrow views had delayed the progress of botanic medicine, some who had originally admired and supported him soon found it
necessary to break from his grasp. "Had he wielded the same influence
for the organization of colleges, that he did in the establishment of his
practice," concluded Anthony, "there might be today a prosperous college in every State in the Union."[3]

A curious phenomenon then occurred within the movement of botanic medicine: botanic practitioners quietly dropped the name Thomsonian and adopted such sobriquets as *reformer* or *medical reformer*,
botanic, *improved botanic*, *independent botanic*, *independent Thomsonian*,
physo-path, and *physio-medical*. The botanic movement also expanded its
materia medica, preferring to identify less with Thomson's sheet anchor
of steam and puke and, instead, administering vaccination for smallpox
and employing botanic medicines opposed by the founder. Increasing
numbers divested themselves of Thomson's bias against formal medical
study and chose instead to establish medical schools and societies built
around the botanic materia medica.[4]

Exemplary of this new emphasis was J. Jackson, M.D., who in the
New England Botanic Medical and Surgical Journal in 1847, took exception
to the class of botanics that served a few weeks apprenticeship in some
of the medical stores and infirmaries of Thomson and then sought to
convince the public of their diagnostic and therapeutic skills. "What a
nonsensical mode of appealing to the public . . . when it is well known,
that Dr. Thomson was never very liberal with his knowledge, that he
laughed at the idea of study at all, and taught that any man of common
capacity, after reading the *New Guide to Health*, was qualified to enter
practice at once." Besides, observed Jackson, for the greater part of the
time, Thomson's students were "consumed in sawing wood, washing
floors and dishes, and packing up medicine, instead of being devoted . . .
to the study of the different branches of the science of healing." Jackson
did not disparage Thomson's system but believed that America required
strong schools and colleges in order that botanic practitioners could
have a thorough medical education.[5]

Defections

The first serious defection from Thomsonism occurred when Horton Howard (1769–1833), a Columbus printer and publisher and an early agent of Thomson in Ohio and the Middle West, authored his own two-volume *Improved System of Botanic Medicine Founded Upon Current Physiological Principles; Comprising a Complete Treatise on the Practice of Medicine* in 1832. Howard formed a dissident group called the "improved botanics," and he started *The Eclectic, and Medical Botanist,* a biweekly journal published between 1832 and 1834. The journal became the organ for his independent botanic thinking, an advocate of greater choice in medical treatment, an official source of rebuttal to criticisms directed at Howard from the *Thomsonian Recorder* (the first periodical marketed in the West in the interest of Thomson's patented system), and a vehicle for advertising Howard's own patent and discussing the merits of his improved system.[6]

Although crediting Thomson with having initiated a much needed reform in the practice of medicine, Harvey D. Little, editor of *The Eclectic, and Medical Botanist* and spokesman for the improved botanics, found his theory "extremely vague, and often erroneous; being founded upon a misapprehension of correct physiological principles." Thomson's system was far from "that desirable state of perfection to which the science of botanic medicine must eventually arrive." In contrast, Little praised Howard for establishing a theory and practice based "upon a new combination of principles, in strict accordance with correct physiology, and in harmony with the . . . operations of Nature, as displayed in the human system."[7]

Howard did not stray far from Thomson, which suggests that he was less a schismatic than a disaffected colleague turned rival. Drawing on the successful marketing techniques of his mentor, Howard employed agents and subagents to sell his own medicines, books, and "improved rights" to practice. He also traveled through Kentucky, Tennessee, Georgia, the Carolinas, and Alabama teaching the principles of the improved system.[8] Thomson, fearing the success of his former pupil, directed his own agents to threaten lawsuits for patent infringement. Howard responded by expressing determination "to defend, to the utmost extent of the law, in any Court of the United States, however distant it may be from my residence, the first suit . . . against any Agent of mine, for the sale of my books, or patent medicines, upon the fallacious ground of its being an infringement of Thomson's patent."[9]

Howard added forty-two plants to Thomson's original materia medica of seventy plant drugs, but his principles and practice of medicine remained unchanged. Like Thomson, he gave no credence to earlier systems of nosology and confidently asserted that they were nothing more than speculative amusements that did little to improve the healing art. Nevertheless, his ideas were surprisingly similar to those of the Philadelphia physician Benjamin Rush (1745–1813), who held that all diseases arose from a general proximate cause and, if curable, were to be treated with a general remedy. Specifically, disease resulted from a diminution of the vital power of the organism, manifested by a failure of strength, a loss of tone to the organs, or a foulness of the stomach and intestines.[10] But unlike Rush, who treated patients with a depletive regimen of bleeding followed by high doses of calomel and jalap, Howard preferred to prescribe herbs that strengthened and gave tone to the organs, cleansed the stomach, and emptied the bowels.[11] "Our remedies are all simple," explained Howard, "as nature herself is simple." Moreover, botanic medicines were harmless. Instead of "preying . . . upon the vital power, and thus contaminating the fluids and destroying the tone of the organs," the botanic materia medica was truly therapeutic in its effect on disease.[12] In concert with other sectarians, Howard urged the proponents of botanic medicine not to "forge their own chains" of prejudice and mystery that had so dominated the "despotism and scientific tyranny" of allopathic practice. They must instead "throw off the yoke of scientific oppression" and begin to "honor [their own] judgments, and do justice to posterity."[13]

Following Howard's death from cholera in 1833, the Thomsonians increased their legal assault on his followers and their beliefs. The improved botanics eventually disappeared from the scene, but not before Howard's book went through three editions, and the executors of his estate (Joseph Howard, John Howard, and D. N. Morgan) sold additional rights to his patent, which had been approved August 25, 1832. Lacking leadership and perseverance, some of the improved botanics returned to the Thomsonian fold; others joined ranks with the eclectics who had already distanced themselves from the Thomsonians, or allied with the growing number of independent reformers who had yet to identify with any particular group or clique.[14]

Other examples of efforts to expand Thomson's materia medica are found in the works of Elisha Smith and Morris Mattson. Smith, a botanic physician from Rochester, New York, began his practice around 1820 and authored one of the first statements of botanic philosophy designed to reach a reading audience beyond the lay public. In 1825, he moved to New Brunswick, New Jersey, and three years later, he established a comfortable practice in New York City. Not to be confused with Elias Smith (1769–1846), the controversial clergyman and early advocate of Thomson's patented system, Elisha served as president of the New York Association of Botanic Physicians, which he founded in 1828, and wrote *The Botanic Physician; Being a Compendium of the Practice of Physic, Upon Botanical Principles*, published in 1830. The book represented an early synthesis of contemporary botanic practice; it expanded the plant materia medica to include several mineral remedies; and it stressed the need for botanic physicians to become educated in all branches of medicine. Smith challenged botanics to become more professional by removing the stigma of the uneducated practitioner from the lexicon of botanic practice.

Like others among the reform botanics, Smith readily admitted his intellectual roots in William Buchan (1729–1805), the Scottish author of *Domestic Medicine; Or the Family Physician* (1769); publicist Robert Thomas (1766–1846), editor of the *Farmer's Almanac* (1792–1846) and author of *A Treatise on Domestic Medicine* (1822); physician and historian James Thacher (1754–1844), author of *The American New Dispensatory* (1813); naturalist Constantine Samuel Rafinesque (1784–1840), who wrote *Medical Flora: Or, Manual of the Medical Botany of the United States of North America* (1828–1830); and Samuel Henry (1769–1843), who wrote *A New and Complete Family Herbal* (1814). But unlike many of his contemporaries, he was not averse to using mineral medications and even surgery when circumstances warranted. Smith's significance came from the fact that he advanced botanic medicine beyond the strict focus of Thomson. His medical society disbanded shortly after his death in 1830.[15]

Morris Mattson (1809–85), physician to the Reformed Boston Dispensary, published *The American Vegetable Practice; Or, A New and Improved Guide to Health, Designed for the Use of Families* in 1841. Initially hired to assist Thomson in the revision of his *New Guide to Health*, Mattson soon had a falling out with his mentor, a situation that resulted in yet another effort to give greater professional focus to the adherents of botanical medicine. In his attempt to denigrate Thomson's significance among botanics, Mattson alleged that the founder's true discoveries were "extremely limited."[16]

Another reformer was John Thomson, one of Samuel's sons, who published *The Thomsonian Materia Medica or Botanic Family Physician* in 1841 in response to Mattson's defection. Although John Thomson sold the book under the name of his father and dedicated it to Benjamin Waterhouse, he actually endeavored to establish botanic medicine on a more authoritative foundation by drawing upon the medical ancients as well as from regulars. A veritable storehouse of terms, pictures, histories, and new plant additions, the book also sought to place botanic medicine on a higher level of intellectual acceptance.[17]

Alva Curtis and Schism

As noted above, the coup of the improved botanics failed to materialize into a permanent organization because of the sudden death of Howard in 1833. Six years later, however, Alva Curtis successfully split from Thomson by establishing his Independent Thomsonian Botanic Society.[18] In contrast to Thomson who explained the purpose and extent of the practitioner's education as "the study of patients, not books, experience, not reading," Curtis encouraged a didactic education that closely paralleled proprietary medical education. He advocated the establishment of colleges and infirmaries in Georgia, Maryland, Mississippi, New York, Ohio, and Tennessee dedicated to the theory and practice of sanative medicine.[19] The independent Thomsonians, in large measure, realized these desires. Over a period of two decades, they transformed Thomson's highly charged mass movement into a school and philosophy of medicine that was quasi-intellectual, boasting a half-dozen medical colleges that borrowed heavily from the symbols of regular medicine.

These changes materialized through a process of slow but determined rebellion within the ranks of Thomson's most ardent disciples. One catalyst for this dissent came from the blind obedience demanded by the movement's founder, which proved too much for even his staunchest followers. However, none of the dissidents could equal the charisma and organizing abilities of Thomson. Curtis, for example, lacked the grass roots appeal that Thomson had so effectively used to dominate reform medicine. Although an effective and popular communicator, Curtis's more bookish approach to medical reform failed to match Thomson's close ties to democracy and his allegiance to the common man. To compensate for this weakness, Curtis used every opportunity to appeal to the memory and achievements of his mentor while pursuing an independent course.

Those independent Thomsonians who extended botanic practice beyond the scope of Thomson's original plan were always ready to applaud the founder's commitment to self-expression and self-government. From their perspective, Thomson had labored hard in the vineyards of medical reform to bring reason out of therapeutic chaos. In honoring Thomson, Charles A. Stafford wrote many years later: "He naturally had a large brain which was only rivaled by Daniel Webster's large head." He was a natural genius, a self-made American who had "the wisdom of a Solomon, with the depth of a Newton, with the logic of a Plato, with the acuteness of observation of a Darwin." He could comprehend the most difficult facts, but remained unencumbered with Greek, poetry, Latin, the mathematics of the college curricula, and the "pet medical theories" of his day. Instead, Thomson went to the "College of Nature" for his schooling and discovered there a universe that was worlds away from that taught by old-school doctors. Thomson's greatest effort at originality was his "intuitive knowledge that the laws of nature are constant."[20]

The independent Thomsonians honored Thomson as the founder of botanic medicine but recognized Alva Curtis as the venerable father of reform medicine's more professional stance. Born in 1797 in Columbia, New Hampshire, Alva was the son of Chauncey Curtis, a soldier in the American Revolution. In 1815, he became a teacher of Latin and mathematics at Great Neck, Long Island, and after three years, used his savings to enroll in a two-year program at Union College. About the same time, he became attracted to medicine when one of his brothers reportedly died from a mercurial treatment. Lacking money to enroll in medical school, Alva accepted charge of the female department of Wenton Academy. During that time, he studied medicine under the mentorship of a Dr. McKelway and discovered what he believed were well-founded objections to allopathic practice.

In 1820, Curtis enrolled in a course of lectures on botany, after which he traveled around the country supporting himself by selling book

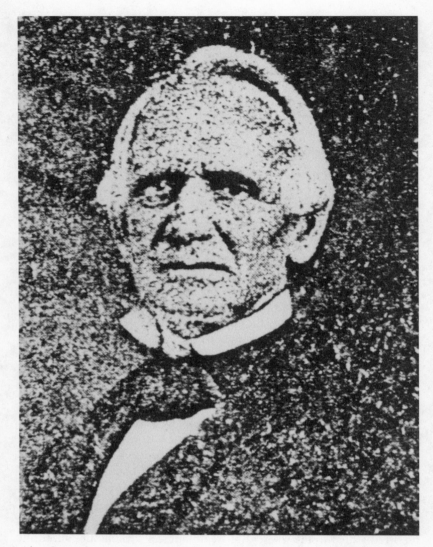

Alva Curtis (1797–1881). From Otto Juettner, *Daniel Drake and His Followers; Historical and Biographical Sketches* (Cincinnati: Harvey Publishing Company, 1909), 111.

subscriptions. From that time on, he accepted botanic practice in place of allopathic principles of treatment. He moved to Richmond, Virginia, in 1821 where he taught language in Mrs. Broome's Female Seminary.

Six years later, he opened his own seminary, and although the evidence is unclear, he supposedly became enamored with the abolitionist ideas of William Lloyd Garrison. In 1829 he married Harriet Ann Carter of Richmond and, during the cholera epidemic of 1832, treated students and himself in accordance with the Thomsonian method. In practicing Thomsonism, Curtis simply availed himself of a movement already rooted in Virginia through the efforts of William Fonerden, a clergyman and botanic healer. Notwithstanding Fonerden's popularity, Curtis soon became Virginia's best-known botanic—a general agent for Thomson's books, patents, and medicines; an organizer of Friendly Societies; an advertiser for the sect's extraordinary cures; a critic of traditional medicine; and an instructor and manager of an infirmary.[21]

Not surprisingly, Curtis's decision to support Garrison and to espouse Thomsonian medicine brought eventual opposition from the community, including the medical fraternity. His actions also resulted in a decline in the academy's enrollments. Forced to close the school, Curtis moved to Columbus, Ohio, in 1834, where he devoted himself exclusively to the practice of medicine and gathered around him a number of students and enthusiastic disciples. In 1835, Curtis replaced Thomas Hersey (1766–1836) as editor of the *Thomsonian Recorder*. The journal was published by Jarvis Pike and Company and initially endorsed by Thomson who utilized it as the official organ of his patented system.[22]

Before Curtis broke ranks with Thomson, he used the pages of the *Thomsonian Recorder* to encourage the licensing of family practitioners (see sample form on p. 34) through the auspices of the branch organizations of the Friendly Thomsonian Botanic Society. These botanic doctors were thus able to enter practice outside the avenue of established medical schools. Of course, many Thomsonians—before and after Curtis's split with Thomson—practiced without a license.[23]

Curtis opened the Botanico-Medical College and Infirmary in April 1836 to instruct others in reform medicine. The school operated without a state charter, and certainly its existence was contrary to Thomson's own bias against the establishment of medical schools; however, it did not lack for students, many of whom had followed Curtis from Virginia.[24] Ever an entrepreneur, Curtis encouraged botanic societies to raise a fund for the education of young men who could be sent to the college. By selecting those "of the best talents and moral principles, and lend[ing] them, without interest, on bond payable when they shall have earned the money (say yearly after they enter practice) so much as they shall need to enable them to prepare themselves well for the work," Curtis thought he had discovered an alternative source of "thorough-bred Thomsonians" to counter the elitist ranks of allopathic medicine.[25]

———— Branch of the Friendly Thomsonian Institute, or the Botanic Society of the United States.

To All Whom It May Concern

KNOW YE that we, the undersigned, Members of the Examining Committee of the ————Branch of the Friendly Thomsonian Botanic Society of the United States, having full confidence in the integrity, sobriety, intelligence and medical skill of Dr. ————— ——————, and more especially being satisfied of his knowledge of the Thomsonian Practice of Medicine, do hereby authorize and empower him, the said Dr. ————— ————— to practice medicine under the right and authority of Letters Patent from the United States, granted to Dr. Samuel Thomson, the 23d day of January, in the year of our Lord one thousand eight hundred and twenty-three.

Given under our hands and seals, at ————, this ———— day of ————, 183—.

In response to inquiries on the school's philosophy, Curtis explained,

On the first of April we commenced the systematic and constant instruction of a Class of young gentlemen, in the true theory and Practice of Medicine. The principles of the science are clearly explained and illustrated, in so great a variety of ways as to fix them permanently in the mind. Our practice affords ample means of exhibiting to students the symptoms of disease, the modus operandi of medicines, and the various and most convenient and proper ways and means of rendering the remedial agents and the curative processes effectual. The science of Botany is familiarly and practically taught in such a manner as not only to acquaint the student with the botanic Materia Medica; but to enable him to examine the whole vegetable kingdom with pleasure and profit. It is illustrated, not merely by books and plates, but by anatomical examinations of the natural subjects, and by oral instructions in the field, as well as in the lecture room. Each student is taught to label and preserve plants for his future benefit. Instructions are given and Lectures delivered on Natural Philosophy and Chemistry. Much attention is devoted to Midwifery, and the forms of disease peculiar to women and children. Anatomy, Physiology and Surgery receive all desirable attention, and the old theories and practices meet their just due, in thorough examination, and comparison with the Botanic.[26]

Curtis used a variety of texts in his instruction, including the works of Thomson and Rafinesque, Benjamin S. Barton's *Elements of Botany; Or, Outlines of the Natural History of Vegetables* (1803), Samuel Robinson's *Course of Fifteen Lectures, on Medical Botany* (1829), articles from the *Thomsonian Recorder*, Amos Eaton's *Manual of Botany, for North America* (1829), and his own publications. He offered students access to his personal library and provided a single classroom for lectures and instruction. Tuition was one dollar per week, plus an additional three dollars for room and board. The course lasted from six to eighteen weeks, depending on the student's background and abilities.[27]

On March 3, 1839, Curtis founded the first state-chartered medical school of the Thomsonian schismatics, known as the Literary and Botanico-Medical Institute of Ohio, in Columbus. The term of the charter was for thirty years. The first class opened with twelve students, and lectures were given over a three-month period. Two years later, because of the distance of Columbus from "the great thoroughfares of travel" and its reputed poverty in dissecting material, the college moved to Cincinnati. There, it regularly changed names (sometimes called the Botanico-Medical Institute, the Botanico-Medical College, or Literary and Scientific Institute) until 1850 when it took the name Physio-Medical College, which it retained until closing in 1880.[28] Since the college neither owned its own building nor purchased apparatus for instruction, the faculty were required to rent facilities for their lectures and furnish their own equipment for demonstrations. The first notable home for the college was Madame Trollope's Bazaar Building, erected in 1828. The college moved into the Bazaar in 1843 and stayed until 1851; it later moved to several other residences, but none had the flair and reputation of the Bazaar, which remained one of Cincinnati's more renowned historic structures.[29]

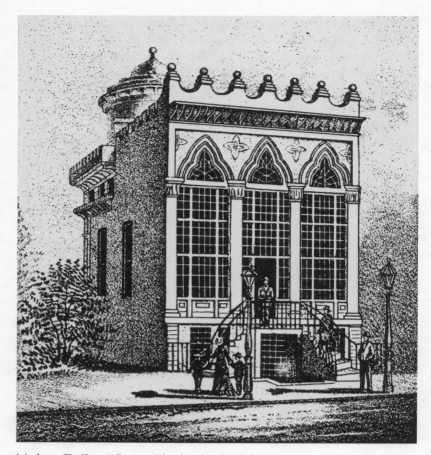

Madame Trollope's Bazaar. The first home of the Physio-Medical College, Cincinnati (1839). From Otto Juettner, *Daniel Drake and His Followers; Historical and Biographical Sketches* (Cincinnati: Harvey Publishing Company, 1909), 109.

Cincinnati proved to be a good choice, and the college soon became the intellectual center for the independent Thomsonians, later known as the physo-pathists in the South and East and the physio-medicals in the Middle West. These appellations did not come without controversy; indeed, the reform wing of the Thomsonians suffered from the effects of regionalism, the lack of an enduring national association, and the fact that botanic reformers seemed less suited by temperament to accepting a single source of authority. As a result, the names *medical reformer, physo-*

pathic, and *physio-medical*, were used interchangeably in the early years following the schism.

Among Curtis's many admirers was Dr. Gideon Lincecum (1793–1874), a self-taught naturalist who was raised on the American frontier and who corresponded with many leading scientists of the day, including Elias Durand and Joseph Leidy of the Academy of Natural Sciences, Spencer Baird of the Smithsonian Institution, Alpheus Packard of the *American Naturalist*, and naturalist Charles Darwin. Born in Georgia, Lincecum moved into the Alabama territory in 1817, then into Mississippi, and finally into Texas. Unschooled except for his own curiosity, he began practicing medicine in 1830, treating patients under the rubric of allopathy and relying on the old school's depletive regimen of bleeding and calomel. Concerned with its fearful effects, he learned botanic medicine from a Choctaw medicine doctor and proceeded to carry two medical bags—one allopathic and the other botanic—and practiced whatever system his patients preferred. He eventually read Thomson's *New Guide to Health* and became an ardent believer in Curtis, Horton Howard, and the reformed school of medicine. Lincecum's correspondence with Curtis spanned more than twenty years; he sent two of his sons, Leonidas and Lucullus, to the college where they learned the basics of reform practice.[30]

In his position as president and professor at the college, Curtis focused his efforts on broadening "Old Sammy's" materia medica of seventy plants; urging a stronger educational grounding in medicine; differentiating the systems of regular, homeopath, eclectic, and physio-medicalism; and advocating equal rights under the law for his school. He appointed assistant lecturers for the school, but reserved for himself the role of principal teacher. Lectures covered anatomy, physiology, surgery, obstetrics, the theory and practice of medicine, chemistry, materia medica, and the general principles of botany. The college's most important course was Curtis's own theory and practice of medicine with which he prepared students to "combat error," "advance truth," and "remove every obstruction to the full, free and universal action of the vital principle." The cost of lecture tickets and access to Curtis's reference library was twenty-five dollars, plus three dollars per week for board, washing, and lodging.[31]

By 1848, Curtis's college had graduated 119 botanic doctors and boasted 83 students. Equally significant, the circulation of the *Thomsonian Recorder* had grown to 2,250 paid subscribers. Curtis remained editor of the journal until 1855 when, under the name of *Physio-Medical Recorder*, he sold it to a colleague and later adversary, William Henry Cook (1832–99), another leading exponent of Thomsonism, who, along with Curtis, established much of the canon of physio-medical thought.[32]

As the reputation of Curtis's school spread, the size of his faculty increased, eventually reaching six. They included Curtis, styled "the Calhoun of young medicine," in the institutes and principles; James Courtney (1804–62) in practical medicine and obstetrics; Joseph Brown in botany, materia medica, pharmacy, and therapeutics; E. Morgan Parritt in chemistry and medical jurisprudence; James A. Powers in surgery; and E. H. Stockwell in anatomy and physiology.[33] Initially, Curtis distributed 70 percent of the proceeds from tuition as salaries; later, after 1848, he arranged to sell each member of his faculty a sixth of the property of the college and the right to equal authority in conducting its affairs. The professors reputedly failed to pay for their rights, but undaunted, Curtis handed over to them the management of the college and its infirmary in order to free himself to travel and lecture on the botanic medical system.[34]

Curtis was anxious to spread his brand of botanic practice even when it wandered into regions of the country controlled by other reform schools. His forays into Boston, beginning in 1848, elicited a sharp response from New England botanics who accused the "Cincinnati Chancellor" of "stooping from an elevated position in the community to accomplish [his objectives] by . . . dishonorable means, and unholy purposes."[35] According to one anonymous critic, the only motive that could be found for his incursion into New England was an "overweening desire of self-aggrandizement."[36] Undeterred by the criticism, he embarked with two of his faculty (James A. Powers and E. Morgan Parritt) on a summer tour of the United States to identify friends of medical reform, awaken interest in the principles of physio-medicalism, and solicit money to place the college "on a level with the best American and European medical colleges."[37]

The faculty and trustees of the Botanico-Medical College, who were beginning to think that Curtis was too authoritarian to suit their purposes, used his absence as an opportunity to separate themselves from his leadership. As soon as he departed on the lecture circuit, they proceeded to reorganize the school.[38] Since the charter for the college was actually a university charter, the trustees petitioned the Ohio Legislature for permission to separate the Medical Department (Botanico-Medical College) from the Literary Department. On March 22, 1851, the legislature granted the petition. The Literary Department, where "gentlemen can better qualify themselves for the study of medicine," remained at the site of the old college on Third Street and was placed under the direction of Curtis and a separate board of trustees. The Medical Department moved to the corner of Western Row and Fifth Street, under the direction of professors E. H. Stockwell, James A. Powers, R. C. Carter, H. F. Johnson, E. Morgan Parritt, and Joseph Brown (who served as dean of the faculty). The Medical Department changed its name from the Botanico-Medical College to the Physopathic Medical College of Ohio and dedicated itself to "innocent medication."[39]

When the medical department failed for lack of strong management, Curtis regained control. In need of resources, he sublet the building as a hotel on terms that he hoped would enable him to sustain the college, and he moved the college's classes into the attic. Several fires, plus the hotel's failure, prevented him from retaining the building. Undaunted by these setbacks, Curtis rented new facilities, resumed his lectures, and hired back those professors who had earlier deserted him. By October 1855, he had built enrollment to forty-two students.[40] However, the bright days of reform were over. According to William H. Cook, who assumed duties as both the chair of materia medica and as dean of faculty, Curtis proceeded to quarrel "incurably" with his colleagues, forcing many of them to leave the school in disgust.[41]

Ever a purist in reform medicine and a convert to physio-medicalism from eclecticism, Cook found the school lacking in proper therapeutic rules, including a thorough understanding of botanic remedies. Determined to correct matters, he proceeded to build a more systematic structure into the curriculum and undertook to analyze the efficacy of the botanic materia medica. Much of this work he later embodied in his *Physio-Medical Dispensatory,* published in 1869. Cook's efforts to strengthen physio-medicalism brought him into early disagreement with Curtis and other faculty in the college who sneered at his drug experiments and surgery, calling them "Cook's hobbies" and avowing that there was little to be added to Thomson's original system of therapeutics.[42] Among his critics was John F. Morey, M.D., of Vandalia, Illinois, who accused Cook of teaching ideas counter to true physio-medicalism. Cook eventually earned the respect of Morey who recognized that, rather than simply following Thomson's strict regimen, it was necessary to enlarge the view and capacity of physio-medical science.[43]

Cook lamented the obstructive tendencies of Curtis and his disciples who, he believed, were anxious lest "the temple of physio-medicalism should be built higher than their heads." If the education from reform colleges was to equal that of allopathic schools and be superior in its use of principles and remedies, then physio-medicalism had to improve its system of therapeutics and not just stand firm with old beliefs.[44] It was time, he urged, for the physios to ask hard questions of themselves. Were the physio-medicals gaining in numbers and in public estimation? Were they being accepted among cultured and scientific men? Were they prepared to meet with educated scientists and physicians and demonstrate the truths of their medicine? Were physio-medicals equal to old-school physicians in the domains of physiology, pathology, chemistry, anatomy, and surgery? Was the spirit of original and independent research strong within the ranks of physio-medicalism? And if not, why not?[45] Unless they addressed these essential questions—and soon—the world would pass them by. Society, Cook warned, "will not allow us to evade [these questions] nor to cover them up; and in these days of wonderful advancement in every department of science, the world will not sustain us if we decline to answer or answer with an uncertain sound." Only if physio-medicalism cultivated a spirit of original research and pushed forward its educational work by enlarging and strengthening its principles with the newest tools of science, could its claims be assured for future generations. By asking these questions, Cook did not imagine the physio-medicalist advocating the acceptance of all new things. "Too many of these new things are at direct variance with the grand principles of Vitality and Sanative Medicine," he wrote, "and are mischievous follies that will soon be swept away." (For discussion of these topics, see chapter 5.) Nevertheless, it was far better to seek truth by pursuing a closer study of science rather than by taking the coward's road of holding back for fear of lending encouragement to error.[46]

Eventually, Cook managed to win over the faculty, but not without creating irreconcilable problems with Curtis who, despite faculty resolutions and warnings from the dean, insisted on placing first-term students in the graduating class. Before long, Curtis was issuing personal diplomas to students who the faculty had refused to graduate.[47] A faculty vote meant nothing to him as he "would over-ride it at his pleasure."[48]

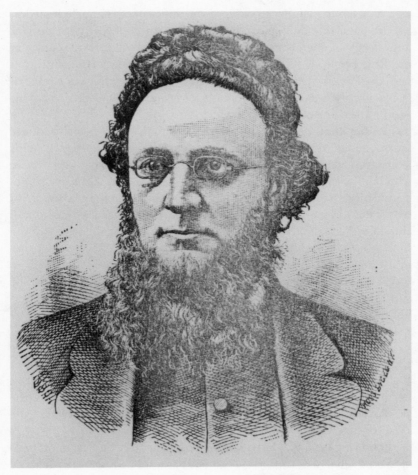

William Henry Cook (1832–99) founder of Physio-Medical Institute, Cincinnati. *Cincinnati Medical Gazette and Recorder* 40 (1881): frontis. Courtesy of the Lloyd Library and Museum, Cincinnati.

Knowing that Cook and his faction were gaining command of the college, Curtis wrote to the board of trustees in January 1858, asking permission to resign his professorship and devote the remainder of his career to traveling and lecturing on reform medical practice. Cook and the faculty refused to accept his resignation "on any other ground than that of positive inability to perform the duties of his chair."[49] Foiled in his attempt at an honorable retirement, Curtis accepted an appointment as professor of chemistry, physiology, and mental and moral science at the Ohio Female College, six miles north of Cincinnati. His connection with the Physio-Medical College remained as before but, to the relief of the faculty, he was removed from teaching and was at liberty to use his pen for the cause of medical reform.[50]

In a matter of months, his connection with the Ohio Female College soured, and in March 1858, he again petitioned the trustees to accept his resignation that he "may retire to the shades of seclusion and rest, to which all pioneers . . . are justly entitled."[51] This time the trustees accepted his request by elevating him to membership on their board. With his reputation saved, Curtis announced his intention to begin a tour of the states.[52] He offered to carry his medical and surgical practice to the four corners of the nation, giving special attention to diseases "peculiar to the fair sex."[53]

Cook and the college faculty took the opportunity to reassure the supporters of Curtis that his resignation would not make the least difference in the future course and management of the institution. The college would remain true to the doctrines of vital force, the unity of disease, the abjuration of all poisons, and the commitment to sanative therapeutics.[54] In point of fact, Cook and the faculty were relieved that the trustees accepted Curtis's resignation since his practice of awarding certificates without faculty approval had done "fearful damage to [the physio-medical] cause [and] more injury than all the allopathists of the land put together."[55]

Following his tour, Curtis returned to the college, and from his position on the board of trustees, continued to award certificates in defiance of the school's standards. Feeling powerless to change the situation, Cook resigned from the college in 1859 and established a rival school a few blocks away. With Cook gone, Curtis resumed full managerial control of the school. By this time, little teaching was done in the college, and when the school's charter expired in 1869, Curtis turned the school into a diploma mill, selling certificates for fifty dollars each. He also devoted his remaining years to writing and revising his books.[56]

One positive legacy left by Alva Curtis was his belated interest in a woman's right to medical education. However, given the timing of his support, which paralleled the expiration of the school's charter and his more nefarious activities in selling diplomas, one should be cautious in attributing any egalitarian motives to his resolve. On the surface, he seemed genuinely sincere, arguing that a woman should have the opportunity to become "anything and everything to which she is . . . adapted . . . provided she does not, in doing so, infringe upon the equal rights of others."[57]

To ensure that medical opportunities were made available to women, Curtis urged that instruction in anatomy, physiology, hygiene, pathology, and the theory and practice of medicine be taught in every school, academy, and college open to women; he further recommended that female medical colleges be constructed and endowed for the benefit of women only. To this end, he solicited gifts for the purchase of grounds, buildings, apparatus, and an endowment for a chair in medicine. There is no record of his success or of the disposition of any monies he collected for this purpose.[58]

In 1880, after a decade of operating as a diploma mill, the Physio-Medical College closed. According to one alumnus, had the school been properly managed, history might well have proved very different for it and for the physios in general. Instead, the reputation that Curtis gave to the institution's last years of existence forced a numbing effect on the botanic reform movement, with many of the college's earlier and respected graduates now all but overshadowed by its new notoriety.[59]

THREE

Years of Challenge, 1839–1859

Given the decided emphasis of American society in the early nineteenth century for individual choice instead of regulation as the preferred public policy, the reform descendants of Thomson moved quickly to capitalize on what they perceived as their newfound strength. Second-generation botanics agreed that in the management of more severe diseases and surgical emergencies, the common man could not gain sufficient information from Samuel Thomson's *New Guide to Health,* Morris Mattson's *American Vegetable Practice,* Horton Howard's *Improved System of Botanic Medicine,* or similar family books on reform medicine. Such understanding could come only from study at qualified colleges with competent teachers. Recognizing this emerging need, reform physicians opened a half dozen medical colleges between 1839 and 1859. The instruction given in these schools followed the principle of aiding the body's vital force to cure disease by "perfectly sanative agents" alone. Only a professional education, the reformers believed, could satisfy the rising expectations of American culture.[1]

Southern Botanico-Medical College

In December 1839, the same year that Curtis opened his Literary and

Botanico-Medical Institute in Columbus, Dr. Lanier Bankston, known to many reformers as the "Curtis of the South," obtained a charter for the Southern Botanico-Medical College at Forsyth, Georgia. The Georgia Legislature assisted the college with a grant of five thousand dollars.[2] In an advertisement published in botanic journals, the college explained its adherence to Thomsonian practice and announced the purchase, for the illustration of surgery and obstetrics, of a French mannequin that separated into 130 different parts and exhibited 1,700 objects in detail. Fees consisted of a matriculation charge of five dollars, a "contingent fee" of five dollars to the chair of anatomy and surgery, and a ticket charge of eighteen dollars to each of the five chairs (M. S. Thomson in obstetrics and diseases of women and children; L. Bankston in physiology and pathology; M. S. Bellenger in anatomy and surgery; Robert C. Bryan in materia medica, therapeutics, and chemistry; and J. Thomas Coxe in the principles and practice of medicine and dean of the faculty). The college's four-month session opened annually on the first Monday in November and concluded on the last Friday of February. The faculty assured interested students that following a rigorous course of subjects and, for a graduation fee of twenty-five dollars, they would receive an "elegant diploma, executed on fine parchment from a large and beautifully engraved copperplate, and in the customary style of the best Medical Institution in the United States."[3]

Prominent reformers who sometimes taught at the college included Henry M. Price and William Fonerden in obstetrics and diseases of women and children; P. MacIntyre in chemistry and medical botany; Isaac Miller Comings in anatomy and surgery; J. Sinclair in materia medica and therapeutics; and George J. Cook in physiology and pathology. In 1857, the college faculty published a text entitled *The Reform-Medical Practice: With a History of Medicine, From the Earliest Period to the Present Time, and a Synopsis of Principles on Which the New Practice is Founded*, dedicated to the powers and benefits of sanative medication. It was subsequently adopted by the Botanico-Medical College of Memphis, Metropolitan Medical College of New York City, and the Physio-Medical College of Ohio. More than eleven hundred pages in length, the book drew from standard works in medical orthodoxy as well as from the writings of Thomsonian reformers, and it presented a full compendium of botanic theories, recipes, and regimens.[4]

One of the early faculty members of the Georgia school was Isaac Miller Comings (1812–89) who, after a somnambulant career in various academies in the South, happened upon Samuel Robinson's *Course of Fifteen Lectures, on Medical Botany* (1829), a book second only in popularity to Thomson's *New Guide to Health*. In many ways, Comings typifies the path of many nineteenth-century botanics. Deciding to pursue career medicine, he apprenticed himself to an old-school doctor but continued to read about Thomsonian practice. When the reform medical college in Georgia opened its doors in 1839, he resolved to matriculate, entering at the opening of its second session in 1841. Concurrent with his studies, he accepted a full partnership in the medical practice of J. Nunnally, one of the college's trustees. Upon graduation in 1842, Comings filled the chair of anatomy, where he remained until 1848 when he moved to the New England Botanico-Medical College in Worcester.[5] In an address before the Georgia faculty and students in 1845, he gave tribute to his Thomsonian origins. "Generation after generation shall pass away, and other names, that are now occupying the highest niche of earthly fame, shall be forgotten, but the name of Samuel Thomson can never be forgotten till that millennium arrives, when pain and sickness shall no more be known."[6]

Comings returned to his former professorship in the Georgia College when it moved to Macon but, in 1852, chose to divide his time between Macon and New York City where he opened a practice and also held a chair at the Metropolitan Medical College. He found time in these years to publish the *Journal of Medical Reform* and, in 1859, moved permanently to New York City where he practiced until his death. His contributions are found in the *Water Cure Journal*, the *Phrenological Journal*, the *Physio-Medical Recorder*, and the *Physio-Medical Journal*.[7]

The school's official journal, the *Southern Medical Reformer*, edited by S. F. Salter, began publication in January 1845, and it boldly proclaimed on its masthead: "Truths that the Theorist could never teach/And observation taught us, we would reach."[8] Edited in later years by H. M. Price and J. Thomas Coxe, the journal advocated three basic principles of Thomson's practice of medicine. The first was a belief in the unity of disease: no matter how varied the causes, or however modified by the organ or tissue which was the seat of the local affliction, disease was in its essence and character still the same. Second, fever, or the pathognomic signs of fever (heat and redness), was not actually the disease but only the evidence of a diseased action. This led to the journal's third principle of watching and following nature in the removal of disease, advocating the use only of medicines that were safe and efficacious in their action and which did not diminish the stamina of life. Based on these principles, the Georgia reformers maintained a regimen of steam and an inverted action of the fluids, namely puking or vomiting.[9]

There was never any love lost between Curtis and the faculty of the Southern Botanico-Medical College. Curtis had refused to promote the cause of the southern college, and in response, the Georgia reformers accused him of being a "monopolizer" and an "aristocrat," governing his college as a "complete monarch and tyrant." The Georgia faculty also accused the northern school of being in league with communism, mesmerism, spiritualism, freesoilism, and abolitionism.[10] For their part, the Cincinnati physios were vexed by the Forsyth and Macon faculty who seemed to pick their quarrels about two or three months prior to the commencement of lecture terms, believing that by attacking a sister institution, they might draw a larger number of new matriculants.[11]

The liberal element within the Georgia faculty (i.e., those botanics who advocated a broader incorporation of therapeutic regimens than stipulated by Thomson) eventually turned to eclecticism and its encouragement to draw from any and every source those medicines and modes of treating disease that proved successful. The eclectics had viewed the canon of medical literature as partly verifiable by experience but mostly unreliable. This meant that eclectics had to enlarge their experience, train their judgment, and decide for themselves, guided always by common sense and decent instincts. When these eclectic views infiltrated the Georgia faculty in 1844, three of the teachers left in protest, and a year later, the institution moved to Macon where it opened as the Reformed Medical College of Georgia. It suspended operations in 1861 because of the Civil War; opened again in 1867; and in 1874, changed its name to the American College of Medicine. It finally merged in 1881 with the Georgia Eclectic College and continued under the banner of eclecticism until 1916 when the school closed for good.[12]

Alabama Medical Institute

Another early physio-medical college was the Alabama Medical Institute of Wetumpka, Alabama, organized in 1844 and composed largely of secessionists from the Southern Botanico-Medical College. The faculty included James M. Hill in anatomy and surgery; O. L. Shivers in theory and practice of medicine; H. Quin in obstetrics and diseases of women and children; W. P. Hatchett in materia medica, therapeutics, and pharmacy; and L. F. W. Andrews in chemistry and botany.[13] Hoping to provide moral support to the new school, the southern students at Curtis's Botanic-Medical College corresponded with Hill and offered their encouragement. "We, as reformers in the healing art, and as inveterate enemies of the old system of scientific poisoning and quackery," they wrote, "feel a deep and abiding interest in the fate of your intended project."[14] Unfortunately, too many of Alabama's botanical advocates preferred to receive their education in the North, forcing the college to close after a single session in 1845.

Botanico-Medical College of Memphis

In 1846, the Botanico-Medical College of Memphis, Tennessee, was chartered with thirty thousand dollars for buildings and apparatus and a faculty that included George W. Morrow in anatomy, physiology, and pathology; T. C. Gayle in institutes and practice of surgery; M. Gabbert in theory and practice of medicine; K. P. Watson in materia medica, therapeutics, and pharmacy; S. R. Jones in obstetrics and diseases of women and children; and W. B. Morrow in chemistry and medical jurisprudence. The annual circular for the college advertised the school as a "pillar of reform" in the South. It boasted an extensive library collection; modern chemical and philosophical apparatus; an excellent cabinet of geological and mineralogical items; an extensive assortment of specimens and life-like drawings of the country's indigenous plants; anatomical and pathological specimens; and various instruments and appliances for the illustration of surgery and obstetrics. The course of instruction lasted four months, with tuition set at eighty dollars, a matriculation fee of five dollars, and a graduation fee of twenty dollars.[15]

Although dedicated to the beliefs of Thomson and the independent reformers, the college followed the path of several other botanical schools by coming under the influence of eclectic thinking. Enamored by John King's concentrated resins and lured by the opportunity to practice medicine in a spirit of liberality, the Memphis faculty turned to the use of concentrated medicines and, in 1859, changed the name of the college to the Eclectic Medical Institute of Memphis before closing

in 1861. Like several other botanic colleges, it was a victim of both
the resinoid craze and the financial consequences stemming from the
Civil War.[16]

The Virginia Institute

On March 8, 1847, the General Assembly of Virginia created a body
politic and corporate called the Board of Directors of the Scientific and
Eclectic Medical Institute, in Petersburg. Its professors included A. M.
Black in anatomy; Charles James Kenworthy in surgery; Wooster Beach
(the recognized father of eclectic medicine in America) in principles
and practice of medicine; E. C. Banning in obstetrics; Henry M. Price in
therapeutics and materia medica; and John Thomas in chemistry and
forensic medicine. The board designated L. J. Kenworthy as dean of the
faculty and Wooster Beach as president.[17] When Beach resigned, Isaac
Miller Comings filled his chair of principles and practice of medicine.[18]
The charter of the institution gave the faculty the power of conferring
the doctorate in medicine on any person "without reference to time
of study, provided the candidate shall have paid for one full course of
tickets, and the matriculation and graduation fees." Along with other
schools, its annual course of lectures opened on the first Monday in November and continued through February. From five to seven lectures
were delivered daily and "in no school in our country is the material for
the prosecution of Practical Anatomy so abundant as in this. It can be
obtained in any quantity, and free of expense."[19] In its circulars, the college gave notice that its professors subjected students to daily examinations, believing that "great benefit . . . derived from frequent inter-
rogation, which serves to impress the knowledge communicated more
deeply upon the mind of the student, and, at the same time, to enable
the teacher to ascertain whether he has thoroughly comprehended it."
Tickets for the course of study cost seventy dollars, not including a matriculation fee of five dollars and a graduation fee of fifteen dollars.[20]
   Although none of the faculty denied the school's botanic purposes,
the institute became a battleground for both Thomsonians and Eclectics. Price, who held the chair in therapeutics and materia medica, experimented with eclectic practices and tried to entice both factions into
some form of accommodation. The efforts proved futile and the institute
reaffirmed its Thomsonian roots until closing its doors in 1851.[21]

Worcester Medical Institute

One of the more notable medical reformers in the New England region was Calvin Newton (1800–1853) of Southborough, Massachusetts. Educated during his primary years by his parents, he enrolled for three years at Brown University where he joined the Baptist church; he then transferred to Union College where he graduated with the bachelor and, subsequently, master of arts degrees. In 1829 he was ordained pastor of the Baptist Church in Bellingham, Massachusetts. Three years later, he joined the Waterville College faculty where he taught for five years, resigning in 1837 to become president of a newly established theological school in Maine. Four years later, he resigned to become pastor of the Baptist Church in Grafton, Massachusetts.[22]

Because of failing health, Newton turned his attention to the study of medicine in the early 1840s and quickly came to the conclusion that allopathy was unsound, if not decidedly dangerous. The reform ideas of Samuel Thomson appealed to him, but he concluded that they did not represent a perfected system. He noted the differences that had arisen between Thomson and his disciples and the direction of medical reform under the lead of men like Alva Curtis, Wooster Beach, Morris Mattson, Elisha Smith, and others. With this in mind, he pursued a course of medical study at the Berkshire Medical Institution (regular) and, upon graduation, joined the Massachusetts Medical Society. Continuing to believe in the need for reform and lamenting the lack of botanical medical schools nearer than Ohio and Georgia, he resolved to start a journal and open an institution that could serve the needs of reformed medical practice in the New England states.[23]

In January 1846, Newton began publication of the *New England Medical Eclectic and Guide to Health*. In the same year, a group known as the Uxbridge Botanic Society employed a Dr. C. W. B. Kidder of Providence, Rhode Island, to give a course of medical lectures. In addition, the society held a convention that, besides bringing together reform-minded botanics, passed a resolution encouraging the establishment of a medical school in Worcester dedicated to reform practice. In the aftermath of the convention, a small group of reformers organized as an informal board of trustees and appointed both Newton and Kidder as professors in the newly formed Worcester Medical Institute.[24] Eventually, the faculty included Isaac Miller Comings in anatomy and surgery; Calvin Newton in physiology, pathology, and materia medica; James M. Buzzell in anatomy and surgery; L. Bankston in theory and practice, and institutes of medicine; and William Fonerden in obstetrics, chemistry, and botany. Later additions included Walter Burnham in surgery and obstetrics; Michael Gabbert in theory and practice; George W. Morrow in anatomy and physiology; Levi Reuben in materia medica and botany; and Henry G. Darling in physiology, chemistry, and botany. As with other reform schools, many of the faculty were academic gypsies, moving from one college to another, teaching a fall term at one and a spring term at another. This explains why college listings so often included faculty from distant institutions.[25]

During its first year of existence, the school entailed considerable debts, covered largely by donations from Newton himself and from John A. Andrews, a local booster of botanic medicine. Within months, Newton assumed responsibility for the school, and in 1847, he and the board sought charter recognition from the Massachusetts legislature. Opposition from Harvard, the Berkshire Medical Institution, and the Massachusetts Medical Society convinced the legislature to refuse the application. Undaunted, Newton arranged for the school to act temporarily under the charter of the Botanico-Medical College in Forsyth, Georgia. Using a legal loophole, Worcester granted diplomas to its students as a branch of the Georgia college. To facilitate the unusual arrangement, Newton changed the school's name to the New England Botanico-Medical College, a change that satisfied those in Georgia who feared the college might not remain dedicated to the principles of medical reform. For those few students who questioned the legality of the degree, Isaac Miller Comings (who held faculty chairs at both institutions) reassured them that the arrangement had been approved by a superior court judge in Georgia.[26]

As part of the agreement, the Worcester college assessed a fee of twenty-five dollars for each degree it conferred, of which five dollars was paid to the Georgia college for expenses incurred under the arrangement.[27] Less than a year later, the Worcester college canceled its agreement with the Georgia college and, instead, arranged with the trustees of the newly formed Scientific and Eclectic Medical Institute in Petersburg, Virginia, to become a branch campus and offer degrees under its auspices. This change stemmed from a decision by the Forsyth faculty to refuse to graduate its Worcester students unless Newton turned over *half* of the graduating fees instead of the five dollars as originally agreed.[28] Under the arrangement which Newton worked out in August 1847, the

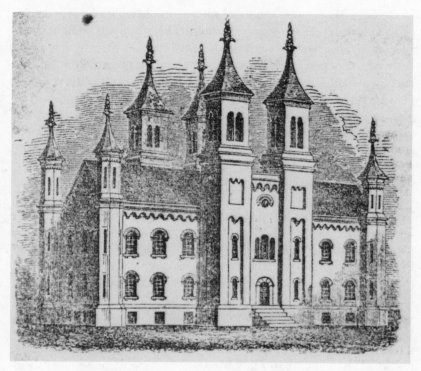

Worcester Medical Institute (1853). From *Worcester Journal of Medicine* 8 (1853): cover. Courtesy of the Lloyd Library and Museum, Cincinnati.

board of directors of the Virginia institute authorized the faculty of the Botanico-Medical College at Worcester to grant diplomas to those persons they considered qualified. For this consideration, the Worcester college paid the treasurer of the Virginia institute five dollars for each diploma conferred.[29]

Newton signed a similar contract in January 1848 with the faculty and board of the Botanico-Medical College in Cincinnati. In this agreement, Cincinnati professor John Kost (1819–1904) accepted a joint appointment on the faculty of the New England college, and both institutions agreed to exchange their anatomical drawings and pathological specimens.[30]

Kost played an important role in the early years of reform medicine, urging his fellow botanics not to become ensnared by the competing terminology. There were those stalwarts who adhered to the appellation of *Thomsonian*, preferring it to all others. This group was small by comparison to those who chose to be identified simply by the term *botanic*. Another sector of the reform movement chose the name *eclectic*, believing it necessary to select and choose what to them appeared the very best plan of medication. A fourth group adopted the name *physo-path* or *physio-medical* (depending on the region), while a fifth group used the more generic term, *reformed medical physician*. On the fringe of these five groups were others who preferred the terms *physio-eclectic* and *hydro-eclectic*.[31] In choosing to identify themselves in so many different ways, the reformers tended to diminish their credibility. They reminded one critic of a "squad of half-intoxicated newspaper boys arguing politics."[32] Kost traced the term physopathy to *phusa*, meaning wind or a pair of bellows, and he doubted whether medical reformers really wanted to be identified with that descriptive. On the other hand, he did not disparage the term *eclectic* for those who wanted to isolate themselves but thought that the simpler term *reformer* would serve the mainstream of medical botanics. The only meaningful alternative to this was *physio*, from the Greek *physis*, meaning nature, which was his second choice.[33]

Among the problems encountered by the New England botanics was a circular sent out by Alva Curtis in 1848 giving notice that the professors of the Cincinnati school would be giving a course of medical lectures in Boston. Fearing unfair competition, the Worcester faculty claimed they alone held true title to the term reform. Struck by the insult, the Cincinnati school responded that the Worcester faculty were "a little too strongly Thomsonians."[34]

In August 1848, Curtis sought to heal the rift by writing Newton and explaining the purpose of his trip to New England. Feigning innocence, he said that his intent all along had been to aid reform medicine rather than to injure the Worcester faculty and its college, but his good intentions had been thwarted by others. "Instead of uniting with you to command the respect and patronage of New England," he wrote, "we were obliged to work alone, to fulfill our engagements to the individuals who met us in Boston."[35] Newton responded to Curtis's olive branch by noting that Dr. John Kost, who once filled the chair of materia medica and therapeutics in the Worcester college, had succeeded to the same chair at Cincinnati in place of H. F. Johnson. "If the other departments [in Cincinnati] are as ably filled as this now is," Newton wrote, "we can assure those students, who may contemplate resorting to the Botanico-Medical College of Ohio . . . that they will . . . receive adequate instruction in the various branches of medicine." With Newton's encouragement, Curtis and his faculty arranged joint appointments with the Worcester school.[36]

Noticing the success of Orran P. Warren, M.D., in obtaining a charter for the New Hampshire Botanic Medical Society, Newton decided to make another attempt at a charter for the college. But instead of seeking strength through unity, he and the faculty wrangled over their identifying names, debated the qualifications for professorships, and, in the process, destroyed much of the public's good feeling toward them by their own internecine squabbling.[37]

To prepare for the college's third attempt in 1849, Newton hired a lobbyist to advance the sentiments of the school. This, plus extensive testimony before a special committee of the Massachusetts Legislature (members included Dr. John Ware, president of the Massachusetts Medical Society; Dr. Henry Jacob Bigelow, the society's former president; and Dr. Henry G. Clark of the House of Representatives), proved successful as both houses of the legislature passed the bill authorizing a charter to the Worcester Medical Institution. It was signed by the governor on the same day.[38]

Once the charter became effective, Newton turned his energies to fundraising, aided measurably by E. Morgan Parritt who the trustees authorized to tour the region on the school's behalf.[39] Parritt's fundraising tour proved remarkably successful and resulted in monies to construct a permanent college on Union Hill, at the junction of Union Avenue and Providence Street, a short distance from "old Harvard, bloated as she is with vain glory, arrogance, and aristocracy."[40] The building accommodated two hundred students: the first floor contained the dean's office, museum, library, and parlor; the second floor housed the chemical laboratory, anatomical cabinets, and anterooms; and the attic served as the dissecting room. Students had access to a medical and surgical clinic under the direction of house physician E. S. McClellan, whose plan of treatment was strictly eclectic, selecting remedial agents based on the nature of each specific disease. In addition to herbal medicines, the clinic offered "water appliances" common in the water-cure (hydropathic) establishments of the country. Professional advice was free, but patients paid for their board and nursing.[41] Students also had use of the

Botanic Infirmary and Bathing Rooms owned and managed separately by Calvin Newton at the corner of Front and Carlton Streets in Worcester.[42] Finally, students could observe surgical operations performed before the class; they were reassured that the anatomical cabinet afforded ample opportunity for investigation, and the school's dissection material was "honorably obtained" and "abundantly supplied."[43] Believing that all medication should be both "innocent and sanative," the faculty encouraged students to consult textbooks eclectically and with discrimination.[44]

The trustees, in keeping with the overtures made by other reform schools, directed the college to enroll one student from each congressional district in the state and to gratuitously admit them to lectures. These recipients paid only matriculation and graduation fees. The board also accepted the hydropathic or water-cure system of medicine as consistent with physio-medical practice and appointed a search committee to find a professor of hydropathy for the college. With the hiring of S. Rogers, M.D., in 1851, the institution formally incorporated hydrotherapeutics into its curriculum.[45]

Tuition at the Worcester Medical Institution was sixty dollars for the first two courses of lectures; subsequent lectures were free. For students who entered with two full courses from another medical college, tuition was ten dollars. For graduates of other medical colleges, tuition was free, except for a matriculation fee of five dollars and a graduation charge of eighteen dollars.[46] These unusual policies reflected the fact that the college encouraged the matriculation of students who had attended instruction in allopathic as well as botanic, hydropathic, and eclectic colleges. The policy, common among sectarian and proprietary schools, not only accelerated the education of medical transfer students, but tempted many schools to become little more than diploma mills.[47]

The medical texts required and recommended for the 1851–52 session at the Worcester college did not deviate to any great degree from other colleges—both regular and sectarian. This was because, in the areas of theory and practice, which accounted for the principal variation among reform colleges, so-called regular schools were equally idiosyncratic in their choice of texts. Of thirty-five books recommended by the Worcester faculty, only six (authors noted in italics), were written by botanic reformers. The balance consisted of allopathic literature.[48]

ANATOMY—Samuel Morton; Sir William James Wilson; Robert Harrison; Joseph Pancoast; Caspar Wistar.

SURGERY—*James M. Hill*; Robert Druitt; Robert Liston; Thomas Castle; Joseph Pancoast.

PHYSIOLOGY—William B. Carpenter; Daniel Oliver.

PATHOLOGY—Auguste-François Chomel; Joseph Williams.

AUSCULTATION AND PERCUSSION—William Wood Gerhard; Henry I. Bowditch.

MATERIA MEDICA—*John Kost*; Jonathan Pereira; George Bacon Wood; Franklin Bache.

THEORY AND PRACTICE—*Horton Howard*; *Morris Mattson*; *Wooster Beach*; Sir Thomas Watson.

INSTITUTES OF MEDICINE—Joseph A. Gallup.

OBSTETRICS AND DISEASES PECULIAR TO WOMEN AND CHILDREN—*Wooster Beach*; Fleetwood Churchill; Nicolas Charles Chailly-Honoré; Jacques Pierre Maygrier.

MEDICAL JURISPRUDENCE—Theodoric Roemyn Beck; Amos Dean.

CHEMISTRY—George Fownes; Edward Turner.

BOTANY—Alfonso Wood; Amos Eaton; Asa Gray.

Candidates for the degree of doctor of medicine had to be twenty-one years of age; attend a minimum of two courses of medical lectures in an established medical college (one of which had to be in residence at Worcester); present testimonials of good moral character and of having been employed three years in professional study from an accredited physician; have a competent literary education; present and defend a dissertation on a subject connected with medicine; and be examined in the various branches of medical study as contained in the course of lectures and in the recommended textbooks. By charter, the trustees were required to confer the degree utilizing "the same rules and regulations which are adopted and required in conferring the same degree by the University of Cambridge, and the Berkshire Medical Institution."[49]

In 1850, a breach developed between Newton and Comings, disturbing the peace of the college and giving "fearful forebodings" to the friends of reform. When the trustees heard the report of the committee charged with investigating the matter, it vacated the chair of theory and practice held by Comings and offered it to Alva Curtis of Ohio.[50] Curtis surprised the trustees by declining the offer and, instead, accepting an invitation to teach a course of lectures in neighboring Connecticut. Insulted by Curtis's decision, the Worcester faculty turned on the Cincinnati reformer, accusing him of unprofessional conduct and of attempting to bring into disrepute a college "where true medical science, the laws of nature, and high unobjectionable Thomsonianism are taught in their purity."[51] Perhaps more importantly, Curtis's impolitic decision turned the Worcester college from its quasi-affiliation with the physopaths of the East and the physio-medicals of the West and placed it more directly under the influence of the eclectics.

As editor of the *Worcester Journal of Medicine*, Newton published the circulars and announcements of both eclectic and physio-medical schools. Increasingly, however, he moved the school toward eclectic thinking, drawn by the successes of eclectic pharmacy (particularly its concentrated medicines) and the school's encouragement of independent, rational medicine. He also joined the National Eclectic Medical Association and reported regularly on the growth of the medical eclectics throughout the United States. "Of the various reform medical institutions now existing in the different states," he wrote, "the teachings of almost all are, at present, in most delightful harmony." The only exceptions he found were at the college at Macon, Georgia, and at Curtis's college in Cincinnati. Since Curtis had not yet resorted to diploma peddling, Newton was probably taking his anger out on Curtis for refusing to accept the institute's offer of a chair.[52]

Despite his increased affiliation with the more liberal eclectics, Newton thought that several of their schools were damaging the cause of reform. He took particular notice of the Eclectic Medical Institute of Cincinnati, which, under the influence of its peripatetic dean of faculty Joseph Rodes Buchanan, had inaugurated a free tuition scheme that was little more than a marketing strategy to steal students from other reform colleges. This unfortunate experiment, Newton explained to his readers, had degraded reform medicine by threatening the livelihood of its most eminent teachers. He had no doubt that the venture was fraudulent; he hoped it would be short-lived.[53] Newton also accused the institute's faculty of using the lancet, mercury, antimony, and other drastic measures calculated to depress rather than sustain the vital powers. He warned eclectics that if they continued on this perilous path, enlightened Thomsonians would turn away from them convinced that "no material alterations can ever be brought about by their efforts in this or any other country."[54]

Newton pointed as well to the fraudulent efforts of eclectics to create professorships. His comments were directed at Wooster Beach who, after leaving Cincinnati, established a medical college in Boston and later in Charlestown. Even though Beach had earned the title "father of eclectic medicine," Newton accused him of having sullied his reputation and the principles of reform practice by establishing a "petty institution" in Boston where students "with only the rudiments of a professional training" could receive the degree of doctor of medicine.[55] Newton claimed that Beach had graduated individuals with less than two weeks' attendance at lectures; worse yet, he had employed as clinical demonstrator a woman whose only experience was as a midwife and nurse.[56]

Months before his death in 1853, Newton was elected president of the National Eclectic Medical Association, which met that year at Rochester, New York. He was also appointed professor of general and special pathology in the Syracuse Medical College (eclectic) and remained an active participant in the affairs of the Massachusetts Physo-Medical Society.[57] With his passing, the trustees of the Worcester Medical Institution reaffirmed the school's adherence to the work of medical reform based upon "no arbitrary, or exclusive, despotic formalities, governed by no overbearing or dictatorial power, but upon the broad, liberal, and democratic principles of medical Eclecticism."[58] Ever so deliberately, the school and its journal moved under the umbrella of eclecticism. Newton was eulogized at the 1854 meeting of the National Eclectic Medical Association where L. Reuben identified him as one of the great "brothers" of eclecticism.[59] His journal, now edited by Frank H. Keley, displayed its official bias when, in October 1854, it announced L. C. Dolley as the winner of the year's prize essay on "The Fundamental and Distinctive Principles of the Eclectic Practice of Medicine."[60]

Along with other reform medical colleges, the institute fell on hard times following the discovery that the concentrated medicines it had adopted from the eclectics were of questionable therapeutic value. John King of the Eclectic Medical Institute of Cincinnati even used the pages of Newton's *Worcester Journal of Medicine* in 1855 to renounce the preparations. "I now wish to call [the] attention of all classes of physicians to a most stupendous fraud which is being perpetuated upon them in relation to concentrated preparations," he wrote.[61] Simultaneous remarks from Edwin S. Wayne in the *American Journal of Pharmacy* and by eclectic John M. Scudder of Cincinnati left little doubt that concentrated medicines were nothing but "unmitigated humbug."[62] According to one disenchanted physio, the Worcester Medical Institution had "put on the eclectic garb" and, like its "apostate sisters of the South," soon regretted the decision. The school subsequently closed in 1859.[63]

Metropolitan Medical College

The charter for the Metropolitan Medical College of New York City passed the New York Legislature on April 12, 1848, entitling its body politic and corporate to operate for fifty years and to conduct a scientific and medical college for the instruction of students in medicine and surgery upon the "reformed botanic system." Signed by the governor July 2, 1852, the school commenced its first course of lectures on March 7, 1853. Fees for matriculation, museum, hospital privileges, and lectures in all the departments amounted to one hundred dollars, plus a graduation fee of twenty dollars. Indigent students were permitted to work out private agreements with the faculty so that their attendance could be secured for less than the established rates. Weekly board ranged from two to four dollars.[64]

Associated with the school in its early years were Isaac Miller Comings in anatomy and surgery; L. Bankston in physiology and pathology; I. N. Loomis in chemistry and botany; J. Thomas Coxe in therapeutics and diseases of women and children; and Henry S. Lincoln in medical jurisprudence. Each of these faculty held appointments at other reform schools and had been recruited at the national convention held in Baltimore in 1852. Even William H. Cook and Alva Curtis of Cincinnati taught during the school's first and second terms. Cook temporarily occupied the chair of physiology and obstetrics, while Curtis held the chair of theory and practice of medicine and materia medica.[65] Joseph D. Friend (1819–89), one of the school's early graduates, and later professor of obstetrics at the college, edited the school's *Medical Journal of Reform*, published from 1852 to 1854. Later he became a strong advocate of free libraries and served in the New York legislature.[66]

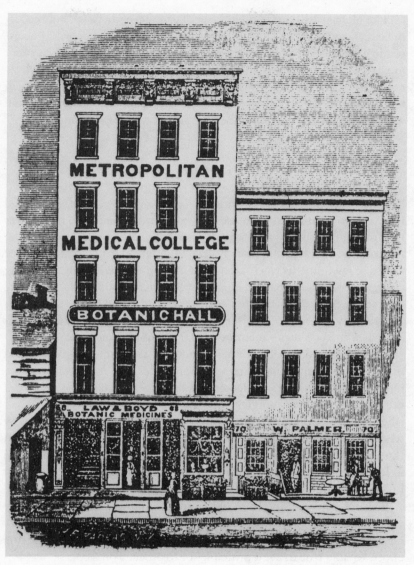

Metropolitan Medical College at No. 68 East Broadway, New York City (1852).
From "Metropolitan Medical College," *American Journal of Medical Reform*
(1852): 360. Courtesy of the Lloyd Library and Museum, Cincinnati.

The physo-paths dominated the college in its early years, but repeating experiences in the East and South, the more liberal eclectics eventually gained control; following the repudiation of their concentrated medicines, the school lost its popular support and closed in 1862. Here, too, as in Curtis's college in Cincinnati, diplomas were sometimes given to first-term students, to some who were not students at all, and to some whom William H. Cook described as "disreputable practitioners."[67]

Retrospect

There were two distinct disadvantages for those reform colleges founded in small towns and villages in the early nineteenth century. The first was the inadequate supply of dissection material, and the second was the lack of adequate hospital and clinical experiences for students. Except for those few students who managed to be apprenticed before attending college, most graduated and commenced practice with only a didactic education. As one observer remarked, the teaching in these schools was "worse than superficial." In some materia medica classes, teachers merely described the botanicals mentioned in Thomson's *New Guide to Health*. "Pharmacy is seldom alluded to, and many of the formulae given would disgrace the pharmacopoeia of a negro root doctor." As for surgery, "we have listened to a course of lectures upon surgery, and the professor did not possess a solitary surgical instrument to exhibit to the class, or wherewith to perform an operation." Instead, he instructed the class by reading from a text. The same situation existed with obstetrics where, in the absence of a mannequin for illustration, "We . . . listened to a course of lectures on midwifery, and the lecturer very kindly read two-thirds of his course from Churchill's *Midwifery*."[68]

The reformers learned the hard way that all of their schools were vulnerable to the more liberal eclectics. The locus for this susceptibility lay at the very heart of the botanic movement, namely, the competing efforts to hold true to a few principles or to proceed on a course of openness to new ideas. Those physios who remained closest to the ideas of Curtis tolerated only minor variations from Thomson's original views. The eclectics, who claimed never to have been disciples of Thomson but only fellow travelers in the realm of botanic therapeutics, appealed to a broader heterodoxy. By the end of the 1850s, the eclectics had successfully absorbed the botanic followers of Thomson in both the East and the South. The incentive for this had come from both camps, but physio faculty seemed especially defenseless before the eclectic wing of botanic reform and the early success of its drug manufacturers. By the end of the Civil War, only Alva Curtis and William H. Cook in the Midwest stood their ground against the siren appeals of the eclectics.[69]

In a moment of honest reflection, physio B. A. Wright, M.D., observed that the early reform colleges had all started with a superior plan of cure that was in accord with natural laws. They assumed unfortunately that its truths were sufficient to fill their lectures to overflowing. Time proved this to be false. The first few physio-medical colleges were either apostates, having turned to eclectic thinking, or were financial failures with managers as "usurpers of power," not willing to allow a fair distribution of authority among the faculty. As a consequence, most of these early colleges collapsed and nearly dragged physio-medicalism with them.[70]

FOUR

Years of Consolidation, 1859–1900

While the physios were attempting to position themselves within the broader landscape of medical education and practice, regular medicine had begun the arduous task of reform. One early sign of this came in 1859 when Nathan Smith Davis (1817–1904) of Chicago, one of the founders of the American Medical Association, sought to institute a five-month course of study with an optional graded curriculum. Having failed to convince Daniel Brainard, surgeon and president of Rush Medical College of Chicago where he was affiliated, to undertake the changes, he and five other physicians founded a medical department in the recently organized Lind University (endowed by businessman Sylvester Lind), dedicated to rectifying the shortcomings of America's medical education system. When, because of business problems, Lind failed to follow through with his expected financial support of the university, Davis and the faculty reorganized the department as the Chicago Medical College and competed with Rush Medical College. In 1869, Davis successfully affiliated the college with Northwestern University. The reforms begun by Davis and the faculty of the Chicago Medical College were subsequently adopted by several other schools, including the St. Louis College of Medicine and Natural Sciences; the College of

65

Physicians and Surgeons, at St. Louis; and the Woman's Medical College of the New York Infirmary, New York City.[1]

In 1871, twelve years after Davis's original initiative, President Charles W. Eliot (1834–1926) of Harvard set out to make the medical school an integral part of the university by placing its faculty on a salaried basis, strengthening admission standards, instituting a graded curriculum, adding new subjects, and establishing a three-year program of nine months each. Following in Harvard's wake, the University of Pennsylvania, the University of Chicago, Syracuse University, and the University of Michigan instituted similar changes. These reforms marked the beginnings of a truly systemic change in medical education as presidents, faculty, and trustees recognized the importance of laboratory facilities; built a firm connection between the university and the medical department; revolutionized the teaching wards in hospitals; and increased the number of faculty teaching basic medical science. German clinical medicine, with its practical implications evidenced by the birth of modern bacteriology, replaced the French clinical tradition with its distaste for experimental laboratory investigation. Forty years before Flexner's famous report, several far-sighted university presidents and German-educated faculty had laid the groundwork for reforming medical education in the United States.[2]

Notwithstanding dramatic changes among the top tier of medical schools, students could still graduate in the 1870s and 1880s by enrolling in a two-year ungraded course of four months duration, avoiding bedside instruction, and taking a minimum of laboratory science. Furthermore, they could obtain a license to practice without ever experiencing a preceptorship or treating a patient. Proprietary colleges continued to operate on a self-support basis, relying on tuition and fees or the sale of lecture tickets, the proceeds of which were divided among the professors in lieu of a fixed salary. In the absence of strong licensing boards and a consensus within the profession as to what constituted an educated physician (i.e., whether medical therapeutics should be founded on empirical clinical observation or experimental laboratory science), these schools continued to flourish in the laissez-faire environment of American society.[3]

The colleges of physio-medicalism were surely not among those elite schools that had begun to lament the disparity existing between progress in the basic sciences and the more stagnant notions of therapeutic rationalism. But neither were they found among those purely mercenary schools whose faculty showed little regard for students beyond the collection of lecture fees. In truth, the physios saw treatment of patients as both their livelihood and the basis of their identity, and they judged any desire to change the state of medicine by offering a new platform of experimental laboratory science as alien and nonsensical. By itself, laboratory medicine was wrongheaded; underlying this prejudice was the belief among physios that medicine remained more art than science. Laboratory experimentation, whatever its claims, represented a redirection of medicine away from the individual patient. It tended to encourage professional distinction in areas far removed from the patient's bedside. If the physios were anything, they were first and foremost believers in family practice.

Physio-Medical Institute of Cincinnati

The Physio-Medical Institute of Cincinnati, under the guidance of dean William H. Cook (1832–99), opened in 1859 to compete with the Physio-Medical College of Alva Curtis.[4] As noted earlier, Cook's estrangement from Curtis had resulted from the latter's selling of diplomas. Cook left Curtis to establish his own college on Fifth Street and Western Row, a few blocks from his former school. There, he propagated the ideas of the independent Thomsonians.

Cook took exception to the divisions among medical reformers, hoping they might find unity amid the divisiveness of their separate societies, colleges, and associations. All true reformers, he believed, should agree to denounce the use of mercury in all of its forms; bloodletting by any means; the whole plan of curing by opposites; and all use of eleven mineral poisons. Provided these principles were embraced, it was wrong for the several factions to reproach each other. Instead, he urged each group to send delegates to the other associations of medical reformers in the hope that some amicable arrangement might follow. For himself, he thought the differences in terminology among the reformers were of little importance. "I am myself an eclectic," he wrote, "but I like the name of PHYSOPATH. . . . It is quite significant of our principles, meaning in its literal sense, a natural affection, or in a more extended sense, a natural mode of removing disease."[5]

The opening of the Cincinnati school came at a difficult time in the nation's history. The term of lectures for 1860–61 closed on January 31, 1861, less than a week before the seceding southern states met at Montgomery, Alabama, to set up a provisional government and less than three months before the outbreak of hostilities. Cook expected a class of forty students to convene at the fall session, but the Confederate victory at the Bull Run (July 21, 1861) sent many of these young men into the army and caused others to stay at home because of the financial gloom spreading over the country.[6] In the September 1862 issue of the *Physio-Medical Recorder*, the trustees announced that the institute would not hold its winter lectures because of the call for volunteers. With the danger of attack by the rebels, "desperate in their determination to possess the provisions and wealth of Cincinnati," prospective students rushed into arms and forced the postponement of the term until October 1863.[7]

Over the course of the war, the Cincinnati botanics gave careful attention to the union's mortality lists, lamenting that they had not been given the opportunity to introduce physio-medical practice into camp life. They also feared the nation was being robbed of its public treasury by the medical monopoly of allopathy, which wished only "to fatten upon the blood and life of the people."[8] Nonetheless, Cook proudly reported that the physios had obtained the position of surgeon to the fourth regiment of reserves defending Cincinnati and had procured places for professors D. McCarthy and W. B. Garside as assistant surgeons.[9]

Following the surrender to General Ulysses S. Grant of Fort Donelson on the Cumberland River, February 16, 1862, Cook offered his professional services free to the Cincinnati branch of the United States Sanitary Commission, promising to provide his own medicines, linen, and competent assistants. When the commission refused to even acknowledge his offer, he made the request to Secretary of War Edwin H. Stanton and accompanied his offer with a petition signed by prominent Cincinnati bankers, manufacturers, and merchants who vouched for his competence. This, too, was ignored. "The silent rejections of my services," he complained in an open letter to President Abraham Lincoln, "are to be traced only to the facts that I do not bleed, or give calomel, opium, henbane, etc.; do not think disease can be cured by opposing the operations of nature; do not think a man's limb should be cut off, when reasonable medication might save it; do not, in short, foreswear my own judgment, and forego all independence of thought and action."[10]

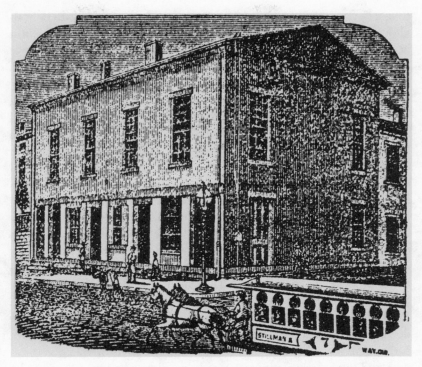

Physio-Medical Institute, Cincinnati (1867). From "Physio-Medical Institute," *Physio-Medical Recorder* 31 (1867): 265. Courtesy of the Lloyd Library and Museum, Cincinnati.

He observed that allopathic surgeons with only a few months of practice were granted commissions while reform physicians who had toiled for years to save limbs and lives were excluded from honorable service. This repudiation of legitimate medical practice did violence to the very soul of free institutions, especially when the sick and dying were denied their choice of medical attendants. Soldiers were forced to adhere to allopathic practice and take medicines and undergo operations without choice or counsel. Even though nearly three million people in the loyal states were friends and believers in reform medical practice, they were forced to submit to allopathic practice. "Now are the deep convictions of these people nothing?" Cook asked. "Must all their hopes, and all their tender feelings, be trampled down, by giving the complete control of the medical department into the care of the very system they have learned to fear?" This situation contrasted sharply with the South, where both allopaths and sectarians treated patients. Cook urged Lincoln to admit at least one physio-medical surgeon in each regiment or hospital to serve as a "check upon the wanton indifference" of allopathic practitioners. Once again, Cook was met with silence.[11]

In his Circular No. 6, issued on May 4, 1863, William A. Hammond, Surgeon-General of the Army, directed that calomel be struck from the Supply Table and that no further requisitions for this medicine be approved by medical directors. Hammond's directive stemmed from evidence that calomel had become "an abuse, the melancholy effects of which, as officially reported, have exhibited themselves not only in innumerable cases of profuse salivation, but in the not infrequent occurrence of mercurial gangrene."[12] His decision brought immediate accolades from reformers who called upon "the benevolent for a donation of rags to absorb the abominable flux from the salivation of the soldiery at Cairo."[13] But the Cincinnati Medical Association (regular) condemned the decision as unproved and libelous and continued to praise the remedial effects of the mercury-based medicine. The following June, a committee of the American Medical Association, consisting of one delegate from each state, convened to consider Hammond's order. Not surprisingly, the committee concluded that the decision had been "unwise and unnecessary" and requested that Hammond modify his order because "the charge of wholesale malpractice [was] unjust to the army surgeons."[14]

The physios, on the contrary, were delighted with Hammond's pronouncement and took special pride in the verses of "Calomel" sung in the sabbath schools in Cincinnati.

Calomel
Physicians of the highest rank—
   To pay whose fees would need a bank—
Have pressed their science, art, and skill
   Into a dose of calomel.

What'er the patient may complain—
   Of head, or heart, or nerve, or brain,
Of fever high, or parts that swell—
   The remedy is calomel.

When Mr. A. or B. is sick,
   "Go for the doctor; and be quick."
The Doctor comes with right good-will,
   And ne'er forgets his calomel.

He turns unto the patient's wife,
   And asks for paper, spoon, and knife;
"I think your husband will do well
   To take a dose of calomel."

He then deals out the fatal grain,
   "This, ma'am, will surely ease the pain,
Once in three hours, at chime of bell,
   Give him a dose of calomel."

The man grows worse quite fast indeed,
   A council's called. They ride with speed.
They crowd around his bed, and tell
   The man to take more calomel.

The man in death begins to groan,
   The fatal job for him is done.
His falt'ring voice in death doth tell
   His friends to shun all calomel.

Now, when I must yield up my breath,
   Pray let me die a natural death,
And bid you all the long farewell
   Without the use of calomel.[15]

Classes at the Physio-Medical Institute of Cincinnati resumed in 1863, and for its fifth annual term of lectures, which commenced November 1, 1864, the faculty included S. E. Carey in theory and practice, obstetrics, and diseases of women and children; D. McCarthy in medical, operative, and military surgery; William H. Cook in botany, therapeutics, and materia medica; George Hasty in general and special anatomy and physiology; and W. Lane in chemistry, toxicology, and chemico-legal analysis. Students paid a matriculation fee of five dollars, seventy-five dollars for the full set of lectures, five dollars for an optional hospital ticket, and an additional twenty-five dollars for the graduation fee.[16]

When Cook sought access for his students at the Cincinnati Hospital (established in 1830 through the efforts of Daniel Drake, M.D.), the Ohio Medical College, which had an agreement to use the hospital as its clinical center, strenuously objected to the request. Unperturbed by the objection, the directors of the hospital responded positively by opening its amphitheater to all medical students for a fee of five dollars (except for the Ohio Medical College students who were allowed to attend free). Feeling betrayed by the decision, the Ohio Medical College faculty rejected the action and asserted the privileges of their original charter. The dispute spilled over into the public press where feelings ran high against the Ohio Medical College and its insistence on a city-approved monopoly. With popular resentment growing, the legislature rewrote the hospital's charter, placing control in a board of commissioners and directing that no college should have exclusive privilege; every student, with the payment of a fee, could attend lectures and walk the wards. Allopathic doctors responded to this democratic action by moving their surgical cases into private hospitals where they could control student access.[17]

The Ohio Medical College lost its monopoly at the hospital, but allopathic influence continued to dominate. The only significant change was that the Miami Medical College, organized in 1852, now controlled staff appointments. Cook insisted that any college "equally honorable in law" should have the right to be represented among the staff; also, paying patients should not be denied their choice of physicians, including those from nonallopathic colleges. Public funds, he argued, "should not be used to sustain one class [of physicians] and to destroy the others. It is not for this that the people pay taxes; and especially will Cincinnatians be unwilling to foot the enormous cost of this hospital, and then have their expensive charity turned into [an allopathic] monopoly." In 1871, the trustees of the hospital accepted Cook's petition to allow the institute's faculty to receive and treat private patients in the pay department on the same conditions as other physicians. Board and nursing was two dollars a day, or one dollar in a ward. Patients who preferred hotel accommodations were directed to the Indiana House at 175 West Fifth Street for two dollars a day, or to Walnut Street House for three dollars a day. Similar concessions were made by Good Samaritan Hospital and St. John's Hotel for Invalids under the management of the Catholic Sisters of Charity.[18]

By the time of its sixteenth annual session of 1875–76, the institute's circular announced enlarged privileges enjoyed by the faculty with the Cincinnati Hospital; five hours of lectures given during each day of instruction; regular class examinations; practical use of the college clinic to familiarize students with the details of bedside medicine; thorough understanding of the materia medica and of the remedial uses of water and electricity; demonstrative teaching adapted to the use of the mannequin and cadaver; and drilling students as a method of teaching habits of exact observation and correct thinking.[19]

Curtis and Cook

For years, Cook had been reluctant to give a full accounting of his feud with Alva Curtis, fearing the damage it would do to the cause of reform medicine. In 1877, however, he decided to clear the air, giving as his reason the passage of the Illinois Medical Practice Act, which empowered the State Board of Health to determine the "good standing" of any medical college whose graduates presented themselves for a license or certificate authorizing the practice of medicine and surgery in Illinois. On the basis of the diplomas presented to the board for its approval, fifty-seven institutions became subject to the board's investigation: forty-three regular schools, ten homeopathic schools, three eclectic schools, and one physio-medical school. The investigation concluded that only fifteen of the fifty-seven schools (fourteen regular and one homeopathic) had established sufficient qualifications for matriculation. The remainder showed no evidence of requiring a preliminary education for their students. Moreover, the board discovered that thirty of the forty-three regular schools, eight of the ten homeopathic schools, and the three eclectic schools conferred the doctor of medicine degree after only two years (approximately twenty-three weeks each year) of study. Included among the schools whose diplomas were rejected by the board were two Cincinnati colleges: the Physio-Medical College of Alva Curtis and the Physio-Eclectic Medical College of William Nicely.[20]

Following its investigation, which included evidence of schools actively selling degrees for a nominal fee, the Illinois State Board of Health published a list of requirements that, if followed, permitted a medical college to be recognized as in "good standing." This included prescribed matriculation qualifications; specific branches of medical science in the curricula; a specified duration and number of lecture terms; student attendance at lectures, recitations, and quizzes; the amount of dissection performed; attendance upon clinical and hospital instruction; the qualifications of the teaching faculty; and the necessary teaching equipment.[21]

The Illinois board eventually accepted the diplomas awarded by the Physio-Medical Institute but, owing to its similarity in name with Curtis's discredited college, had delayed approval in the mistaken belief that the institute was little more than a diploma mill. To resolve matters, Cook invited the president of the board to visit the college and to satisfy himself as to the school's educational philosophy and the quality of its program.[22]

Soon after the Illinois board gave its approval to the institute, Cook went on the offensive to remove any further stigma of the schools operated by Curtis and Nicely. He also publicized information on the notorious diploma-mill operations of William Paine and John Buchanan in Philadelphia and of Curtis's friendship with them. During the 1870s, both Paine and Buchanan had openly sold diplomas. Their fraud was so egregious that one newspaper published the names of more than seven thousand individuals who had received the doctor of medicine from Buchanan alone, including 300 who had received diplomas as physio-medicalists. Curtis, according to his former dean, had visited both men in Philadelphia and, on returning to Cincinnati, joined forces with William Nicely. Both Curtis's Physio-Medical College and Nicely's Physio-Eclectic Medical College offered to make available "good diplomas" for the price of fifty dollars to any student who had failed to graduate from Cook's institute.[23]

Physicians who had earned their graduation honorably from the Physio-Medical College up to the time of Cook's resignation in 1859, were tarnished by Curtis's actions in subsequent years. "Fallen and disgraced by its own acts, so low that men outside the profession cannot recognize its diplomas," wrote one distraught alumnus, the new college had become a "blot and taint on the very name of physio-medical."[24]

According to Cook, the "dark stain" of dishonor that Curtis, Nicely, Paine, and Buchanan had brought to reform medicine represented a "willful betrayal of trust." The high hopes born at the start of the reform colleges had been killed by the actions of these men; their defections from the principles of reform had opened the way for medical laws directed against reform practice.[25]

Occasionally, critics vented their anger at Cook for attacking this revered pioneer in medicine.[26] Undaunted, Cook accused his former colleague of conducting a college without trustees, without faculty, and without a charter, and of willfully swindling the public with his dishonest sale of bogus diplomas. "All the trouble between Dr. Curtis and me started in that one action," he recalled. This singular treason had brought terrible damage to the cause of the college and to physiomedicalism.[27] Curtis had sullied the name and reputation of physiomedicalism by using the authority of the state as "a screen for swindling the people out of their lives."[28]

> Whatever of good Dr. Curtis has done, let it stand; but it is much less than supposed, and was always mixed with his quarrels. His diploma-selling of the last twenty years has been nothing less than an outrage and a blight. When his trustees resigned in 1861, their charter became absolutely void. Every document issued since then in the name of that charter, is a fraud and worthless. This he knew; and never denied it when I wrote him this fact in 1870. Some good men hold his documents; but they are disgraced by the open sale of his papers to hundreds of farmers, mechanics, clerks, and others who are totally without a medical education. The most profound ignorance could get his "diploma" for money. Such sales are a fraud on the State, a fraud on the simple men who buy them, and a profound swindle on the public. Curtis's diploma operations make him the sport and the contempt of all honest men, and I do not aim to carry any share of that contempt for him.[29]

Cook also used the editorial department of his journal to publicly expose those making requests to him for honorary professorships as well as petitions from Methodist ministers to be extended the courtesy of a medical degree (including an offer to trade land for an honorary diploma).[30] He was not embarrassed to report this correspondence since deans at most medical schools received similar requests, a situation that spoke to the traffic in diplomas and to the temptations that faced marginal colleges looking to defray the costs of their operations.[31]

Cook insisted that no state should grant a license to practice medicine until it was satisfied with the competence of the applicant. For this reason, he supported the right of the state to examine individuals who offered themselves to the public as physicians. This power was affirmed by Judge R. C. Pitman of the Superior Court of Massachusetts and by Associate Justice Joseph P. Bradley of the United States Supreme Court.[32] "But examinations on all points where the schools differed should be left to the schools themselves," reasoned Cook, "and no man should be forced to submit his views to the judgment of other schools. This would be a manifest outrage on the rights of private judgment."[33] Accordingly, Cook resented the power claimed by the Illinois State Board of Health and the equally aggravating fact that the governor had refused to place a physio-medical representative on the composite board. Cook threatened to take his case to the Illinois Legislature, urging that all examining and licensing powers be remanded over to the separate incorporated medical societies. He favored the power of examination and licensing to remain with the Illinois board only if *all* philosophies of medicine were equally represented on the board.[34]

School Management

Cook's institution possessed an element not found among many sectarian schools: its faculty never apostatized. Instead, they united in their faith and principles and taught a more definitive plan of medical practice than ever before taught by reform predecessors. The college, however, was not without problems. Its one significant weakness was organization, having been chartered with a dean who was also president, secretary, and treasurer. This meant that disagreements between Cook and an individual instructor usually ended in the termination or resignation of the faculty member.[35]

Unlike most other proprietary colleges where faculty held seats on their governing boards, Cook deliberately separated faculty from the business side of the college. To achieve this, he secured as trustees for the college successful businessmen, manufacturers, wholesale merchants, and bankers dedicated to the philosophy of physio-medicalism; he allowed no physicians on the board. The trustees received no pay for their labor but gave freely of their time and influence. They also solicited donations to support the college. Like deans of regular schools, Cook recognized that the income derived from college tuition was inadequate to support the full cost of medical education. This made it essential to add to the financial basis of the school through concerted fundraising activities.[36]

This organizational arrangement was decidedly different from the typical stockholder form of ownership that Cook was convinced could no longer support a quality medical program. Under that financial structure, professors earned a specified yearly wage and the remaining income was divided among the stockholders. Since stockholders demanded a return on their investment, there was always a tendency to "pinch down the faculty till none but fourth- or fifth-rate can be afforded." When this happened, Cook felt there was no inducement to maintain high scholarship, and the school itself acquired a reputation for meagerness of instruction.[37]

Believing that the better medical schools would have to rely on fundraising to augment tuition revenues, Cook inaugurated a financial plan that directed all monies raised by subscription to be used only for buildings and apparatus, leaving the faculty to meet their own expenses from lecture tickets. Cook insisted that the faculty have nothing to do with the subscription fund; this arrangement left the trustees free to manage the school's physical plant and finances without interference. This action insulated the trustees from possible manipulation by one or two professors while, at the same time, it gave them the authority to ensure that the faculty taught according to strict physio-medical philosophy. To accomplish this, the trustees retained the power to hire and fire faculty according to the best interests of the college. Having secured a board of independent means, responsible principally for the financial integrity of the college, Cook believed he had insulated the institution from the types of internecine disputes that had destroyed so many earlier reform schools.[38]

The arrangement had the grudging support of the faculty who, forced to depend on ticket subscriptions for their salaries, wisely chose to consolidate their several departments to reduce administrative costs.[39] In 1875, however, the faculty anticipated that a new building as well as more modern apparatus would be available for the opening of the next session. When the forty-five students and faculty learned to their dismay that funds were not forthcoming, they took upon themselves the task of raising $3,500 to renovate the existing structure. To their surprise, the trustees refused to authorize Cook to receive the money or to superintend the work. As a result of the impasse, a breach opened between the trustees and the college. For their part, the trustees felt that the institute need not modernize its curriculum and facilities and that any decision to reform or renovate the college resided in their own able hands. Cook, on the other hand, concluded that physio-medicalism would stand a better chance of success if it proceeded more quickly down the road to reform.

Other matters also took shape in the ensuing years, including the realization that physio-medicalism required a larger population base from which to draw students. Added to this, Cook desired a city where the faculty could control their own hospital wards and enjoy a broader sampling of disease pathology. With these added reasons, Cook closed the institute at the conclusion of the 1884–85 session and moved with several of the faculty to Chicago where he opened the Chicago Physio-Medical Institute. Of course, the decision to leave Cincinnati was not a unanimous one. "To many of us, who have been students of that institution and received our degree from its faculty," wrote one discouraged alumnus, "the untimely demise of our Alma Mater is a matter of deep regret, especially as we believe she died from inexcusable neglect on the part of her friends."[40]

Physio-Medical College of Indiana

The Physio-Medical College of Indiana organized in Indianapolis in 1873. Its founder, George Hasty, had read medicine at the age of twenty in the office of a Dr. Joseph Weeks. After two years apprenticeship, he entered the Physio-Medical Institute at Cincinnati and graduated in 1860. He then joined Cook and the faculty for several years before moving in 1872 to Indianapolis where he developed a thriving general practice. A year later, he opened the Physio-Medical College and edited the *Physio-Medical Record* dedicated to the cause of reform medicine. During the early years of the college, Hasty filled several of the chairs himself and, at the same time, occupied the duties of dean, secretary, and treasurer. As

the school became financially stable, he confined his teaching to anatomy and surgery until 1881 when he succeeded S. E. Carey as chair of
theory and practice.[41]

Stalwarts of the school included Andrew Wallace (1816–92), president of the school's board of trustees, who considered himself a lifelong
member of the reformed camp in medicine.[42] Another supporter was
B.B. Turner (1851–93), a graduate of the Physio-Medical Institute in Cincinnati in 1875 and of the Physio-Medical College of Indiana in 1887,
and an active member in the American Association of Physio-Medical
Physicians and Surgeons. Yet another was G. N. Davidson (1829–93) who
as a youth had worked for various farmers in Ohio, learned the brick-
layers trade in 1853, and then began medical study under Professor S. E.
Carey, M.D., of South Fincastle, Ohio. He attended the 1856–57 session
of the Physio-Medical College of Ohio and practiced medicine until his
enlistment in the Union Army. However, like other sectarian doctors,
the Union army denied him a medical commission. After the war, he returned to medicine and practiced for twenty years. He was a stockholder
in the Physio-Medical College of Indiana and a member of its original
faculty in 1873.[43]

One other early supporter of reform medicine in Indiana was Oliver
Perry Stone (1822–82) who grew up in New York and, at the age of seven-
teen, made his way to Winchester, Indiana, where he married, taught
school, and later practiced law. A firm believer in Christianity and the
Democratic Party, he was also a staunch supporter of physio-medicalism
and relied on Curtis's published lectures as the sole medical authority for
his family's health. When the Physio-Medical College of Indiana formed,
he became one of its founding members, subscribing liberally in its stock
and serving as secretary to its board.[44]

The college graduated ten to twelve students annually, including at
least one woman in each class. Its sixteenth session in 1889 was the
largest in the college's history, with nineteen students. Its graduates came
from Illinois, Iowa, Minnesota, Missouri, Nebraska, New York, Ohio,
Pennsylvania, and Texas. The seventeenth commencement exercise in
1890 even included students from Norway, Sweden, and Scotland.[45]

Like other reform schools, the Indiana college extended to women the
opportunity to continue in the role of family healer but, in truth, women
were less numerous in later years than they were earlier. Ironically, as
the medical education system faced the cold reality of much-needed

Annual Announcement of the Physio-Medical College of Indiana, at Indianapolis. From *Physio-Medical Journal* 19 (1893): 13. Courtesy of the Lloyd Library and Museum, Cincinnati.

reform, women physicians became the first casualty, forced into taking a more modest role in the delivery of health care.

The adoption of a four-year program (including one year reading with a preceptor) in 1891 and the addition of histology, microscopy, and sanitary science to the curriculum caused many to fear the school's demise due to a decline in enrollment.[46] This concern seemed all too real when the nineteenth annual commencement exercises at Plymouth Church in Indianapolis conferred the doctor of medicine on only three graduates. Following this brief enrollment decline, however, the numbers of graduates returned to their previous average.[47]

Until 1891, the college occupied fourth-floor offices in the Hubbard building at the southwest corner of Meridian and Washington Streets. In September 1891, the college moved to the upper floors of a building on Indiana Avenue, three squares from Washington Street and one square north of the State House, where it occupied six rooms—office, classroom, library, parlor, and anatomy rooms. Instruction was principally didactive, consisting of six lectures each day, except for Wednesdays and Saturdays when students attended clinics at the City Hospital. In addition, clinics were held each Tuesday at the college where faculty brought interesting cases from their private practices to benefit the students. The library contained current medical works as well as bound journals and writings from the early days of reformed medicine. Its collection also included sets of anatomical charts; pencil, pen, and crayon drawings of the body; oil paintings representing various pathological conditions; and works of the faculty. A museum on the premises contained French mannequins, skeletons, casts, and specimens of morbid anatomy.[48]

Applicants for admission were expected to demonstrate good moral character and provide evidence of having received either a diploma from a literary or scientific college or a first-grade teacher's certificate. Lacking these credentials, applicants had to show proficiency in the branches of a common English education by means of an oral examination before a committee of the faculty. Finally, the college required students to complete twelve months of reading under a preceptor before they applied for admission.[49]

Candidates for graduation had to be at least twenty-one years of age; give satisfactory evidence of good character; show no inclination to use alcoholic liquors in "any quantity"; enroll in three or more courses of lectures; attend hospital clinics and receive clinical instruction during three college terms; pursue the study of practical anatomy under the supervision of a demonstrator; complete at least two courses in practical chemistry; undergo a written examination in each branch of medicine taught in the college; and pay all fees.[50] From the time of its initial graduating class of 1874 until 1890, the college graduated 184 students with the doctor of medicine.[51]

In 1894, the college purchased new quarters at North and Alabama Streets (formerly the Girls Classical School) where it also opened a free dispensary to provide students with clinical instruction. The only requirement for clinic patients was that they bring a letter from some "reputable citizen" certifying they were financially unable to pay for treatment.[52] Firms such as C. H. Stimson and Co. of Newark, Ohio; Wheeler Chemical Co. of Chicago; H. M. Merrell and Co. (eclectic) of Cincinnati; and William Auterwreith of Cincinnati contributed equipment and drugs.[53] The dispensary was small, both in space and in clientele, serving only 125 patients in a five-month period.[54]

By 1900, the college, known among supporters as the "mecca of physio-medicalism," had a teaching force of twenty-nine (principally practitioners who served as adjunct faculty to the college), and offered a four-year program of twenty-six weeks each. Fees were sixty-five dollars each term, and enrollment in the 1900–1901 session was thirty-four, with nine graduates.[55]

By the 1904–5 session, after thirty years of operation, the college boasted a four-year graded course of seven months, a competent and progressive faculty, modern chemical and bacteriological laboratories, and excellent (?) hospital advantages. The first year of the four-year program was devoted to the principles of physio-medicalism and the remaining three years to the practical application of its principles. Course fees for the year were seventy dollars and total enrollment was thirty-two students, with nine graduates.[56] When botanic practitioners in England announced in 1904 their intention to open a school of botanic medicine in Southport, the college offered to waive tuition for those who intended to become teachers in the new school.[57]

In 1906, the college trustees purchased the buildings and campus of the former Northwestern University at College Avenue and Thirteenth Street. Throughout the following summer, construction crews rebuilt and repaired much of the college, putting in a new steam-heating sys-

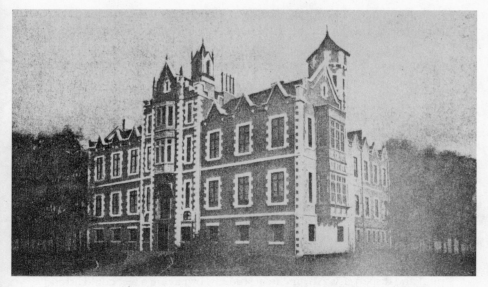

Physio-Medical College of Indiana, Indianapolis (1904). From *Physio-Medical Record* 7 (1904): frontis. Courtesy of the Lloyd Library and Museum, Cincinnati.

tem, a new lighting system, cabinets, and technical apparatus. The north auditorium was installed with elevated, theater-style seating, and the dispensary was completely rebuilt and fitted with surgical cases and operating tables; a room for holding pharmacy supplies; stereoscopical equipment for illustrating lectures; and a full line of ophthalmological apparatus. The old biological hall was redesigned as an operating theater, seating seventy-five students, and Joseph M. Thurston, a member of the faculty, donated a full set of microscopes to equip the new hall of biologic sciences. Finally, the college developed a registration system to maintain medical and surgical records; patients who entered either the dispensary or hospital were given identification numbers to ensure consistency in patient records. This made it easier for students and faculty to make comparative studies of both the pathology and the results of patient treatment.[58]

When the Council on Medical Education, a committee established by the American Medical Association, began to inspect all medical colleges, recommending some for "immediate execution," and others with probation or good standing, the physios found themselves seriously disadvantaged. The Physio-Medical College of Indiana wrote to the Indiana State Board of Medical Registration and Examination in 1907 complaining that the council's inspection had not been carried out in a spirit of fairness and justice. What particularly incensed the college faculty was the council's allegation that the school was deficient in clinical instruction. The college argued that the American Medical Association had been responsible for the very condition of which it complained since regulars in the state had refused to allow physios the opportunity to use the city hospital and dispensary to give clinical and hospital instruction to their students. In an age when both the laboratory and the hospital had become significant sources of therapeutic knowledge, the limited use of this important agency had weakened the physios' professional legitimacy.[59]

All physicians who were not members of the Marion County Medical Association (regular) were denied professional privileges at the city hospital and dispensary. Any medical student, by paying a fee, could attend the amphitheater and clinics at the city hospital; but since physio faculty lacked staff appointments, they were compelled to turn both their patients and students over to regular physicians. The same applied to the patients of homeopaths and eclectics. Because of this injustice, the Physio-Medical College requested the state board to disregard the council's evaluation. "Were it not for these discriminations," the faculty contended, "there never would have been cause for criticism on this point, and when these discriminations are removed, that moment will the clinical opportunities of our students be above any required standard."[60]

The lack of staff appointments in municipal hospitals was only one of the problems facing the physios. Faculty who divided their time between private practice and teaching had little opportunity to conduct the business of the college. This predicament affected all proprietary schools—both regular and sectarian—that relied on adjunct rather than full-time salaried faculty. Responding to this dilemma, in 1906, the Indiana college changed its management structure, hiring C. H. Howland Sherman as its business manager. With the encouragement of the officers, faculty, and board of trustees, Sherman took over the day-to-day management of the college.[61]

In the same year, the college announced the establishment of a sanitarium and hospital under physio-medical management, to be known as the Indiana State Sanitarium. This was the first institution of its kind in Indiana under the direct supervision of the physios, who promised strict adherence to sanative medication. Located on property owned by the school at College Avenue and 14th Street, the hospital offered its operating room and amphitheater for use to the college faculty and students in return for free rent.[62]

The college also adopted a plan to sell stock with a par value of ten dollars per share and to use the monies to equip the hospital. The trustees expected patient fees to support ongoing hospital costs and pay dividends on the stock sold; similarly, student tuition and fees were expected to support the expenses of the college. The trustees also announced their decision to name the school's medical departments for donors willing to place the college upon a more secure endowment.[63]

When these efforts failed to realize their intended outcomes, the trustees looked to one last option. Unable to match the higher admission standards and improved curricula demanded by the country's leading medical reformers, and in the absence of university- and hospital-based affiliations to support the rising costs of laboratory science and clinical medicine, the trustees inquired whether the School of Medicine of Indiana University might entertain a merger of their two institutions. The trustees sought to have their students transferred to Indiana University and, if possible, to have a department of physio-medicalism maintained within the School of Medicine. Receiving no encouragement from university administrators, the trustees closed the doors of the college in 1909. The only concession made by the university was to give students in the failed college the option of transferring as new matriculants.[64]

Miscellaneous Schools

There were various short-lived schools such as the Curtis Physio-Medical Institute of Marion, Indiana, that incorporated in 1881. Henly James was president of the institute and David B. Snodgrass its dean of faculty and founder. James also served in the Indiana General Assembly. The first class graduated in 1882. Upon obtaining new articles of incorporation on January 16, 1893, the school moved to 711 North Tennessee in Indianapolis where it graduated classes in 1893 and 1894. Snodgrass also listed his permanent residence at the same address. In

1894, the school moved to 827 North Illinois in Indianapolis (offices of Snodgrass and McKinsey, physicians) and listed Snodgrass as dean and president; Laura Snodgrass as secretary; and Charles S. James as treasurer. In late 1894, the school returned to Marion but, failing to receive recognition by the Indiana State Board of Medical Registration and Examination, closed in 1900.[65]

The Twentieth Century Physio-Medical College of Guthrie, Oklahoma, incorporated in 1900. The school's dean, H. Warner Newby, advertised "correspondence departments" at Union City, Michigan, and Hatfield, Pennsylvania, where for ten dollars, one could purchase shares in the Twentieth Century Health Association. According to published brochures, these shares empowered their bearers to obtain diplomas permitting them to practice medicine "anywhere in the United States." The school was identified as fraudulent, and the state revoked its charter in 1904. Finally, there was the Thomsonian Medical College of Allentown, Pennsylvania, organized in 1904. Its actual affiliation to physiomedical theory remains unclear, and there is no evidence that classes were ever held.[66]

Postscript

Beginning in the 1870s, the pressure for medical reform came from inside and outside the nation's university-based medical schools. Within universities, leadership started with a few visionary presidents but moved quickly to an inner core of German-educated professors in preclinical subjects who held Ph.D. degrees and who advanced an exciting new ethos in research. Outside the universities, leadership came from state licensing boards and boards of health; the Association of American Medical Colleges; the Carnegie and John D. Rockefeller foundations; and from the American Medical Association's Council of Medical Education.

At the other end of the reform movement were the physios who, despite their pretensions, never quite felt at ease with the expectations of the new age. Having prided themselves in their native roots and herbs, and in a commitment to a domestic practice based on a regimen of kindly medicines (their assumption being that botanical medicines were more naturally assimilated by the body than mineral medicines), they were in no position—intellectual or financial—to manage the changes that medical reform demanded. With the possible exception of William H. Cook, most physios viewed laboratory science and experimental medicine as foreign and elitist, and only grudgingly did they incorporate these components into the curricula of their schools. However, their inability to build a strong financial base and their continued admission of students who lacked preliminary education, including work in the basic sciences, precluded any hope that the quality of their instruction—or the quality of their students—would improve. The physios struggled unsuccessfully to provide the additional staff required for laboratory-based education; no doubt they would have preferred to have been left alone to exist on their own terms and to change at their own speed. But this luxury was not theirs to enjoy.

Even into the late 1880s and 1890s the physios continued to discuss how best to identify themselves. Many concluded that none of the various names expressed the full measure of the school's reform-mindedness. Some of these same people pointed out that the old school's use of the term *regular* had, in effect, implied that anyone out of step with allopathy was out of step with true medical science. Responding to this perceived impediment, some physios suggested using the term *nature's natural physicians;* others recommended a change in their name to the *regular sanopathic school* of medicine and surgery.[67] Using the word regular in this manner would deny allopaths their monopoly of the term. Still others preferred the term *sanopathy* as a more accurate description of the school's preference for kindlier medicines.[68] In the end, however, most stayed with the term *physio-medical* or the shortened *physio,* believing that Thomson's followers were known by too many different names, and one more, however deserving, would prove detrimental to the success of the movement. All agreed that physio-medicalism represented that element of Thomsonism that had become "cultivated, improved, and advanced." It was medicine "in harmony with all the functions of life."[69]

Vitalism and the Materia Medica

During the second half of the nineteenth century, American physicians found themselves in the middle of a contentious debate involving the opposing philosophies of vitalism and materialism. For most protagonists in this debate, the modus operandi of their remedial agents depended on the particulars of their philosophy of organism. "It may seem a far cry from a discussion of what is life to what to do for a typhoid case," observed C. E. Woodruff, M.D., in 1911, "yet every single remedial measure is directed toward a vital phenomenon; consequently, common sense dictates that we should learn what is meant by the word 'life,' for we should not be ignorant of the very thing occupying our whole time. Prolongation of human life is the sole purpose of our professional existence, and it certainly behooves us to know what we are prolonging."[1]

The concept that living bodies contained within themselves an active force that differed from anything possessed by nonliving matter was the starting point for much of reform medicine in the nineteenth century. For vitalists, life represented a new and foreign principle imposed on the materials that constituted the body. In essence, a "directing element" or "force," not under the control of the laws of either physics or chemistry, was resident in living matter. Some interpreted this force to be latent in the materials themselves while others implied the existence of a "soul," or external force, that acted on the body. Life had a dynamic element, inaccessible to human understanding despite known laws that governed the organic and inorganic worlds. In other words, vitalism was a philosophical concept that interpreted causation as a force independent of natural science; a certain "something" existed in living bodies that was not present in nonliving bodies.[2]

Opposed to vitalism in all its various forms was the concept of the body as a mechanism. For the nonvitalist, or materialist, the phenomenon known as life consisted of activities with properties that were subject to the same laws of physics and chemistry as the properties and actions of inorganic bodies. In other words, life could be understood in terms of the processes already revealed by the study of lifeless matter. In this view, the living organism was a machine whose activities were both directed and predictable.[3]

Vitalism and the Physio

The theory of vitalism, as taught in physio-medical colleges, made little pretense of avoiding theological issues, much less metaphysical questions. Throughout the history of botanic medicine, the faculty of physio-medical colleges maintained an obvious and direct connection between the philosophy of vitalism and the practice of medicine. In fact, physios frequently likened themselves to early Christians who offered a "first step" in the solution to the problems of life.[4] They accused regulars of having gravitated inexorably into materialism by denying the proposition of a supreme governing force in the body and arguing instead that life resulted from the simple molecular arrangement of matter. Melville C. Keith, one of the principal physio theorists in the nineteenth century, called the vital force the "life power," or the "spirit from God," and he argued against the "erroneous assertions" of biologist and philosopher Ernst Haeckel (1834–1919); physicist, anatomist, and physiologist Hermann Helmoltz (1821–94); naturalist Charles Darwin (1809–82), and the rest of the "infidel tribe of so-called wriggling scientists." If it were true that blood is life, then, argued Keith, life was the same "force" as the "Spirit." "If this is true, that in this set of atoms dwell the Life

Force, then it will be true that in these atoms, we have the Spirit which goes to God, when the body is dead. If this is true . . . then we have, in our blood, the Spirit of God, who has given us this Life—this Spirit—or loaned us this Life or this Spirit."[5]

The physios enthusiastically joined in the vitalistic debate, identifying themselves both as heirs to the German physician and chemist Georg Ernst Stahl's (1660–1734) principle of *anima* and as opponents of the physio-chemical theories of Joseph Priestley (1733–1804) and Antoine Laurent Lavoisier (1743–94). The science and practice of physiomedicalism was "not the gift or invention of any man or company, nor succession of men," observed Alva Curtis. Instead, it was "the eternal truth and good, science and art of God, and His inestimable and unequaled gift to all who will thankfully receive it and properly apply it."[6] According to the advocates of reform medicine, Samuel Thomson had rediscovered evidence promulgated earlier by Stahl, reviving vitalistic theory and vital force as the law that governed and explained every physiological action witnessed in the living organism.[7]

Among the physios, the faculty of the Physio-Medical College of Indiana were by far the most articulate spokesmen for the philosophy of organism. Joseph M. Thurston, who held the chair of histology and pathology at the college, placed physio-medical theory directly within the context of man's origination as explained in Genesis. He argued that the sciences of anthropology and biology and the "penetrating powers of our magnificent microscopes" failed to give humankind a better explanation to the question of life force.[8] True, the microscope enabled the scientist to understand the *process* of development, but it did nothing to challenge the belief in a special and immaterial force that moved matter. The origin, nature, and destiny of man's inherent life force remained a mystery. At best, scientists could only study its manifestations in and upon living matter. It was important, then, to understand that the living organism was neither a machine run by physics, nor a motor run by an electrical force, nor even a laboratory under the domain of chemical formulae. Rather, the living organism was the "legitimate realm or sphere of action of vitalism." Vital force operating through bioplasm was the only phenomenon of life.[9]

The Indiana college held a steady course through its thirty-six year history, basing its educational system on a bedrock of vitalistic principles. According to its 1883–84 annual announcement,

In therapeutics, the teaching of this College recognizes the physiological condition of the elements of the body as that from which all
vital manifestation emanates, that any deviation in the body from
a physiological state of the solids or fluids gives rise to abdominal
manifestations, the continuance of which must sooner or later produce organic change, or a pathological condition. The processes or
steps by which this change is accomplished is recognized as pathological; therefore, the basis of pathology in this school differs from
that of other schools which regard the change in structure as the
pathological condition.[10]

At the forty-fourth annual convention of the Indiana association of
physio-medicalists meeting in Indianapolis in 1906, Thurston presented
a resolution intended to counteract the dangers of materialism. "The
time has come," he announced to the assembled members, "when we,
as a body of medical reformers, must face the issue and fire the first
gun in the greatest war that the world has ever known . . . for God's
sake and humanity's weal." Specifically, he condemned the scholarly
and scientific works of Darwin, Haeckel, and biologist Thomas Henry
Huxley (1825–95) for advocating a mechanico-biology and a chemico-
physiology. This trend, according to Thurston, had infected all but the
physio-medical colleges, which, alone among modern medical schools,
continued to affirm vitalistic theories. "Not a medical college in the land
except physio-medical colleges but are seeking . . . to forge the chains of
fettered thought."[11] In order to press the issue, Thurston presented to the
physios the following resolution: "Resolved . . . that the doctrine of vitalism as opposed to the souless idea of mechanico-biology . . . is hereby
officially acknowledged as the fundamental basis of the theory and practice of physio-medicalism."[12]

Not all the Indiana physios were as convinced as Thurston that
vitalism and Christianity were the dual sources for the philosophy of
organism and the practice of physio-medicalism. C. A. Stafford, M.D.,
professor of the institutes of medicine at the Physio-Medical College,
attempted to stress the intellectual contributions of Darwin, suggesting
that the English scientist had "emancipated the mind of man from the
bondage of superstition and fate" by directing attention to the physical forces of nature. "Any student who can study Darwin's works, and
not see life dignified and broadened," he remarked, "could sit in a park

among pleasant flowers and beautiful scenery and declare that life has no beauty."[13] For Stafford, the theory of evolution did not attack the Bible; in fact, it "has no conflict with religion." Science had nothing to do with the authenticity of the Bible; it dealt instead with the discovery of the laws and principles of the physical and physiological nature.[14]

Stafford was not alone in his feelings. Physio J. S. Byers, M.D., of Noblesville, Indiana, maintained that the Bible was "comparatively valueless as a textbook in matters of science."[15] Accordingly, he preferred that the principle of vital force be relegated to private belief rather than remain the official basis of physio-medicalism. "Theories based upon metaphysical conceptions of vital force . . . are now rapidly fading before the brilliant light of modern science," he wrote. In effect, the theory should be regarded as "nothing more than a clumsy and injudicious attempt to bolster up a false and tottering system of thought." He urged his fellow physios to honestly acknowledge their ignorance "and patiently wait for further developments in science to reveal the facts which we arrogantly assume to understand."[16]

Notwithstanding the efforts of Byers and Stafford to separate religion and science and to place the curriculum of the Indiana college on a more empirical basis, colleagues accused them of joining in a conspiracy that included philosopher Herbert Spencer (1820–1903) and other agnostics who rejected the truths of biblical Christianity. For the stalwarts of Christian medicine, the writings of Spencer and the comments of Byers and Stafford represented an attempt to introduce rank skepticism into what they accepted as the truths of revelation. Exemplary of this attitude was Jacob Redding, M.D., who accused his two colleagues of willfully undermining physio doctrine. "There is an impassable gulf between organic and the inorganic that so clearly distinguishes the one from the other," noted Redding, "that the most stupid investigator cannot but recognize the fact if he will honestly and conscientiously seek for the truth as it is in nature." Unfortunately, he observed, Byers and Stafford preferred to ignore the facts of nature and reject all knowledge imparted through divine revelation. Indeed, they had greedily accepted Spencer's assertions of "atheistic authority and bombastic assumption."[17]

The debates surrounding the philosophy of organism caused serious rents within the college and between the faculty and practicing physios. In an effort to minimize the damage created by the feud, editor George Hasty of the *Physio-Medical Journal* explained to his readership that the debate was not a foreboding of bad times for the college. "The physio-medicalists of Indiana are made of different stuff than that which can be knocked to pieces by such a discussion," he wrote. "There is no 'Cook and Curtis' quarrel in it and none such will grow out of it." His best advice to both factions within the college was: "Just keep cool, gentlemen, [and] no fractures will occur."[18] Nevertheless, he admitted publicly that the college had squandered too much of its time on the issue of vital activity "to the exclusion of other matters."[19]

Over and over again, the physios postulated, retreated, and argued the nature of vital action, vital force, and vitalism. Its essential conditions, its elements, its destruction or disturbance, and its functional actions consumed much of their writings—both among themselves and against others. Through it all, they attempted to demonstrate a seamless fabric of thought from the sect's earliest days. Although they admitted to certain imperfections in Thomson's views, particularly the belief that most diseased conditions could be treated with cayenne pepper, sweats, and lobelia emetics, they retained the vitalistic beliefs of both Thomson and Curtis, holding that these ideas had lost little of their original relevancy.[20]

Sanative Medicines

Since vitalism was the first principle of physio-medical practice, it followed that vital force, and not the physician, healed disease. True, physios must sometimes "lead" vital force, but they could never "supersede or usurp its legitimate province." This meant working with vital force, not against it; aiding the *vis medicatrix naturae,* or the healing power of nature, not hindering it; using sanative (supportive) therapeutics, not toxic agents; sustaining and guiding vital action *(vires vitales sustinete),* not destroying it; and relying on repletion, not depletion.[21] Like the homeopaths and eclectics, the physios attempted to reinstate the theory of *vis medicatrix naturae,* which originated in the teachings of Hippocrates and had been resurrected in the seventeenth century by the Flemish physician and chemist Jan Baptiste Van Helmont (1577–1644). The theory postulated that the true relation of medicine to the human organism was one of "cause," not power. Its presence "occasion[ed] vital power to behave unlike what it otherwise would." Thus, for example, medicinal tonics did not impart any special power to the organism or add to the total of the organism's vital power; their use occasioned only a change or manifestation of vital power, a change favorable to nutritive accumulation.[22]

Medicines were a form of matter *acted on* by the bioplasm (the form upon which the life and functional activity of the cell depended) and integrated into it as vital energy; in no sense was its power or energy independent of the tissue elements. True medicines aided the restive and eliminative efforts of vital force by helping restore the normal physiological condition; the bioplasm of the tissue unit converted medicine into energy, thereby changing the functional action of the bioplasm.[23]

The physios also rejected the belief that "specific" therapeutic agents existed in any real sense. In this regard, they were remarkably similar in thinking to both the eclectics and the homeopaths (i.e., specificity did not exist in the therapeutic agent but in the scientific administration of remedies to specific disease conditions). For example, physios did not seek a specific medicine for syphilis; rather, the proper method of treatment first ascertained the specific tissue state and then the "conditions of functional aberrations or symptom-complexes."[24] Likewise, in kidney disorders, the physios knew of agents that caused elimination of urine. This, they argued, was due to the "inherent law of bioplasmic selection" or preference of the tissue unit for certain substances. A diuretic agent such as buchu leaves entered the circulation and was directed by the force of bioplasmic selection to the kidney unit bioplasm, which appropriated its helpful constituents. The bioplasm determined the preferences and needs of the organism; it was "the organizer and builder of the vital domain, the instigator of all functional performances in health and disease, the selector and distributor of all nutritive materials . . . the prime resistive, eliminative and reconstructive force [and] the supreme moving, instinctive intelligence in all therapeutic remedial influence."[25]

In choosing their medicines, the physios relied heavily on lobelia, capsicum, and the vapor bath—all considered sheet anchors of Thomsonism. While they expanded the materia medica, its list of medicines remained well within the contours of Thomsonian practice. Admittedly quick to point out the crudities and errors of Thomson, the physios never lost sight of the medical principles introduced by his system.[26] Since the inherent mission of vital force was to preserve and repair the organism, the physician's responsibility was to imitate the efforts of vital force in treating disease. This meant that drugs such as opium, morphine, cocaine, alcohol, arsenic, and strychnine were contraindicated as the "hydra-headed monsters" of drug medication.[27] All poisons injured the tissue unit; no amount of skill could impart "a curative power to an agent that God has stamped with a power to destroy."[28]

As late as 1903, the physios accused regulars of using 107 poisons in their daily practice. These included twenty-seven combinations of phosphorus, five of strychnia, forty-seven of mercury, twenty-five of opium, and fourteen of arsenic. When regulars responded that a little poison was sometimes a good thing, the physios retorted that the property of matter was constant; "what is an inherent characteristic of any substance is continually the same and is impossible to change while the matter itself is unchanged." A poison retained its essential nature for all times and was forever in a condition to kill living matter. "No man's skill," reasoned F. O. Broady, M.D., in 1903, "though he be a demi-god in the brilliancy of his powers, can change the tendency of alcohol, arsenic, opium, strychnia, belladonna, aconite . . . to destroy each its own peculiar form of tissue according to its special power."[29]

Physio Pharmacy

The early botanics refused to purchase their medicines from regular pharmacies for fear of adulteration. They also objected to the use of Latin in prescription-writing because of its implied secrecy. Instead, botanics tried to control their own drug trade by either making their own medicines or purchasing them direct from wholesale botanic firms. Among the early botanic wholesale and retail druggists were John Thomson (son of Samuel Thomson), New York City; J. T. Gilman Pike, Boston; Drs. J. and Benjamin F. Abbott's Botanic and Thomsonian Dispensary, Boston; Wilson's Thomsonian and Botanic Laboratory, Boston; Godfrey Meyer and Company, Columbus, Ohio; Ward Sears and Company, Baltimore; John Burns's Milford Thomsonian Depot, New Hampshire; Westerfield Pharmaceutical Company, Dayton, Ohio; and D. L. Hale's New England Thomsonian Depot and General Herbarium, Boston.[30]

Following the decline of Thomsonism, the physios lacked sufficient numbers to sustain their own distinctive drug trade. Not surprisingly, they turned to eclectic and regular druggists who advertised in physio-medical journals and who offered a long line of herbal and concentrated preparations. As noted earlier, the physios' reliance on eclectic medicines brought themselves and the eclectics to the brink of extinction. Having been lured by the more liberal thinking of the eclectics and having affiliated with their resinoid craze, most physio colleges that organized their therapeutic practices around these medicines failed to maintain their credibility with the public. This, plus the impact of the Civil War, brought most of the physio-medical colleges to collapse.

Those few schools that survived continued to depend on eclectic or regular pharmaceutical companies for their preparations. Among eclectic druggists, the products of Lloyd Brothers, Pharmacists, Inc. of Cincinnati (formerly H. M. Merrell and Company) were highly recommended to physios everywhere. The reformers also purchased herbs from B. Keith and Company, New York City; Lambert Pharmacal Company, St. Louis; H. C. Luyties, St. Louis; C. H. Stimson and Company, Newark, Ohio; Amick Chemical Company, Cincinnati; Listol Chemical Company, Chicago; Fowler and Wells Company, New York City; Neat-Richardson Drug Company, Louisville; Clinton Pharmaceutical Company, Syracuse, New York; F. D. Hill and Company, Cincinnati; Abbott Alkaloidal Company, Chicago; Jacob S. Merrell, St. Louis; Coolidge and Adams, New York City; and a physio-medical druggist named C. T. Bedford from Indianapolis. The Bedford Drug House supplied physios with pure drugs using standard physio-medical formulas. The company also served as agent for the "green drug" preparations of the William S. Merrell Chemical Company (eclectic) of Cincinnati, which sold an assortment of specific tinctures along with corn silk, saw palmetto, black haw, echinecea, black cohosh, cactus, passion flower, cotton root bark, fringe tree, and stone root.[31]

Parke, Davis and Company (of Detroit, Michigan; New York City; and Kansas City, Missouri) sold drugs to both regular and unorthodox doctors and introduced a number of botanical remedies that the physios praised as sanative, efficient, and valuable. These included coto bark, used as an astringent in diarrhea and dysentery; tonga, a Fijian remedy for neuralgia; and lippia Mexicana, an expectorant. The reformers also praised the pharmaceutical firm of Eli Lilly and Company of Indiana because of the care its employees took in selecting drugs that were pure and fresh.[32] "Honesty, industry and energy has made Mr. Lilly the pill man of the country," remarked the editor of the *Physio-Medical Journal* in 1881.

Advertisement of C. T. Bedford, for physio-medical druggist. From *Physio-Medical Journal* 16 (1890). Courtesy of the Lloyd Library and Museum, Cincinnati.

Lilly sold any number of sugarcoated pills for the physio-medicals, including Ague Physio-Medical, Apocynin Compound, Cohosh Compound, Lobelia Compound, and Podophyllin Compound.[33]

Herbal Remedies

However grateful the physios appeared to industrial pharmacy for the preparation and sale of botanic medicines, they never fully accepted the lack of companies devoted exclusively to their needs. Many, too, had felt betrayed by the eclectics and their overzealous production of concentrated preparations that had entered the market without sufficient investigation. As a result, numerous physios refused to compromise their principles, preferring instead to prepare their own medicines. "I say save your money, and time, and patients, and make your own preparations from the drugs that you have handled yourself," advised Melville C. Keith, M.D., in 1887.[34]

Gathering and preserving medicinal herbs, roots, and barks required knowledge of the proper seasons, judicious selection, and careful processing. Annual roots that grew from seed each year were gathered just before flowering; biennial roots were gathered in the fall of the first year or early in the spring of the second. Triennial roots were collected in the fall of the second year or spring of the third year; perennial roots were collected either in the fall after the leaves and tops began to die or in the spring before they began to grow. After the roots were collected and before they dried, workers washed and trimmed the extraneous material. They then cut the roots into small pieces and spread them out to dry in an airy place or in sunshine, careful to prevent their becoming wet. When fully dried, the roots were packed in jars, boxes, or barrels, according to their quantity, and were placed in an airy room. Leaves were gathered at the time of flowering, dried with the same precautions as roots, and preserved in a similar manner. Barks were gathered in spring or fall, carefully dried, and preserved in a fashion similar to roots and herbs. Flowers were collected when about to open from the bud, or in a state of full perfection, carefully and quickly dried in shade, and preserved as the others.[35]

John Albert Burnett listed thirty remedies as the most useful and popular among the physio-medicalists in the nineteenth century. These

FINE PHARMACEUTICALS.

ELI LILLY & CO.,

MANUFACTURERS OF

Gelatine Coated Pills, Sugar Coated Pills,

FLUID EXTRACTS AND ELIXIRS,

36 AND 38 SOUTH MERIDIAN STREET, INDIANAPOLIS, IND.,

And 314 Delaware St., Kansas City, Mo.

Sugar Coated Pills of the following Prescriptions by Physicians of the Physio-Medical School, sent by mail on receipt of price, postage paid:

AGUE, Physio-Medical ....50c. per hundred, $4.50 per 1000
        Chinoidine.... ... .2 grs.
        Capsicum .... ¼ gr.
        Lupulin.......... ... ... ¾ gr.
        Ol. Peppermint .. . .1-16 gr.

APOCYNIN COMP ....50c. per hundred, $4.50 per 1000
        Apocynin.... ... . ¼ gr.
        Leptandrin... ... . ¼ gr.
        Podophyllin.......... .... ½ gr.
        Ampelopsin........................ .....1-16gr.
        Oil Capsicum... ... ... '.. ....1-16gr.

COHOSH COMP., 3 grs... ... ... 40c. per hundred, $3 50 per 1000
        Powd. Black Cohosh ....1 gr.
        Powd. Helonias..................... . . ..1 gr.
        Powd. Cauloplyllum ....1 gr.
        Ext. Scullcap ....q. s.

CATHARTIC COMP., Physio-Medical..... ... . 35c. per hundred, $3.00 per 1000

LOBELIA COMP., 3 grs................. .... 40c. per hundred, 3.50 per 1000
        Powd. Lobelia Seed.................. ....1 gr.
        Powd. Capsicum ....1 gr.
        Powd. Ladies Slipper........ ....1 gr.
        Ext. Boneset ....q. s.

PODOPHYLLIN COMP. (Eclectic) .... 45c. per hundred, $4.00 per 1000
        Podophyllin..... .. .. ⅛gr.
        Juglandin... .... 1-16 gr.
        Leptandrin.......... ....1-16 gr.
        Macrotin. .... 1-32 gr.
        Oil Capsic .... 1-32 gr.

General List of 1000 Pharmaceutical Preparations sent free on receipt of address.

ELI LILLY & CO.,

INDIANAPOLIS, IND., and KANSAS CITY, MO.

Advertisement of Eli Lilly and Company for physio-medical physicians. From *Physio-Medical Journal* 6 (1881). Courtesy of the Lloyd Library and Museum, Cincinnati.

included lobelia, capsicum, bayberry, chionanthus; an antiperiodic made by taking fluid extracts of gentian and hydrastis, cascara, salicin, myrrh, and simple syrup; tincture myrrh compound; Thomson's composition; neutralizing cordial; scutellaria; ascelepias; dioscorea; stillingia; crawley; sodium chloride; euonymus; fleasbane; calcium lactophosphate; cimicifuga; sodium salicylate; cactus; magnesium sulphate; iron ferrocyanide; iron sulphate; zinc oxide; polemonium reptens; amphiachyris dracunculoides; echinacea; corn silk; iron salicylate; and zingiber.[36] Until quinine was included in William H. Cook's *Physio-Medical Dispensatory* in 1869, it remained on the index of non-sanative poisons.[37] Still, many stalwarts refused to accept quinine and substituted hydrastis canadensis as the best general tonic.[38]

Other popular remedies included castor oil, wormseed oil, anise oil, and tincture of myrrh for a vermifuge; valerian root, ginger root, cinnamon bark, anise seeds, prickly ash berries, and oil of sassafras as antispasmodic aromatic drops; poplar bark, golden seal, bayberry, columbo root, capsicum, and cloves for bitter tonic; mandrake root, black root, blood root, gamboge, lobelia seeds, and cayenne as vegetable cathartic pills; and mayweed flowers, smartweed, bitter archangel, bittersweet, wormwood, and cayenne pepper as nerve ointment. As an alternative to opium and its derivatives, the physios often drew upon the works of botanic Horton Howard who recommended such substitutes as blue cohosh, mullen, bugle weed, cokle burr, greek valerian, twin leaf, and yellow poplar.[39]

For fever, particularly if the patient lived in "hygienic ignorance," the physio-medicalist recommended that the entire perspiratory apparatus be "thoroughly antisepticized." A steam or vapor bath, followed by "a good old-fashioned hot water and soap scrubbing," softened the accumulations in the glands, encouraged perspiration, and rendered the skin less susceptible to bacteria. The physician followed this regimen by frequent sponging with boiled soft water to which various salines, alkalies, or acids were added. Patients were then given caullophyllum and viburnum as ganglionic stimulants; asarum and xanthoxylon frax as capillary stimulants; and cola acuminata or erythroxylon cola for the central nervous system. Physios also prescribed buchu and juniperus as diuretics.[40]

The treatment of consumption elicited special attention by the physios who, like the regulars, found the disease to be particularly life-threatening. Both regulars and physios agreed that the prospect for recovery from consumption depended upon the individual's constitution and the habits, past and present, that contributed to its hold on the victim. If, for example, the disease had become established in an individual with a strong hereditary tendency to the disease, the prognosis was poor indeed. If, on the other hand, the affection seemed more accidental, they offered hope under the proper management of disease.

Regulars recommended that consumptive patients spend as much time as possible in the open air; maintain a regimen of exercise and a diet of easily digested foods; seek a climate that was dry (Minnesota, Colorado, California, or the sunny Mediterranean); take cod-liver oil with meals and opium before sleeping or to relieve the cough; use antimony, ipecacuanha, or squill for expectoration; and sponge frequently with vinegar to relieve perspiration. In contrast, the reformers administered leptandra, hydrastis, iris, or euonymus, combined with disorea, zingiber, capsicum, or zanthoxylum for the lungs; decoctions of tamarack or pine bark for the throat and chest organs; and slippery elm, gum arabic, or comfrey, combined with lobelia herb, capsicum, and licorice root to keep the air passages moist.[41]

In their effort to identify the cause of phthisis, the physios concluded that any habit or condition that devitalized the system and bankrupted its vital force furnished a fertile soil for the disease. To this end, they warned against masturbation, excessive venery, spermatorrheal and leucorrheal discharges, prolonged nursing of children, tight lacing, and poor ventilation. They also condemned belts and recommended suspenders for men, and they warned women to avoid corsets or elastics to hold up their stockings. Clothing for both sexes should be suspended from the shoulders and not from the hips. Patients were to avoid feather beds, sleep only in well-aired apartments, exercise by walking or riding in the open air, and obtain eight to twelve hours of sleep each night. The physios urged a diet of plain foods, including well-cooked grains; raw and stewed fruits; pure milk; garden vegetables (except the Irish potato and tomato); small portions of beef and mutton; occasional use of fish and fowl; and the avoidance of tea, coffee, and chocolate. Finally, they prescribed vapor and water baths, frequent glasses of water, and enemas.[42]

Unlike Thomson and his immediate followers, the physios opposed the use of alcohol in their medicines and, instead, recommended liquid syrups or pills if water did not suffice to extract the plant's true virtues.[43] "From all the evidence before us from Noah down to the present," observed A. H. Baird in 1882, "alcohol has cursed every family, tribe and nation, directly or indirectly, and the thousands of articles discovered for medicines have but increased its use, and following it is an increase of drunkenness, premature deaths, all of which clearly proves that medicated alcohol is not inert but however masked . . . is a fiend infernal."[44] Similarly, the physios opposed the use of tobacco, coffee, and tea, claiming that they "injuriously affect the morals of society by leading to habits of meanness."[45] According to Melville C. Keith, author of *Childbirth and the Child* (1888), male alcohol users and tea drinkers were habitual losers of semen through nocturnal emissions.[46] So sure were physios of alcohol's destructive ends that they made its prohibition a formal part of the graduation requirements for their medical colleges. Not surprisingly, many physios were active members of temperance societies. Exemplary of this was Catherine Ann Masseker, wife of William H. Cook, who obtained her early medical training in her father's botanic drugstore, and who became a leader in the temperance movement.[47]

Knights of the Lobelia-Pod

Lobelia (otherwise known as emetic weed, Indian tobacco, puke-weed, gagroot, eyebright, vomitwort, and bladder-pod), named in honor of the Flemish botanist and physician Mathias de Lobel (1538–1616), was a plant six to twenty inches in height, with numerous small, delicate blue flowers. The plant was annual in the warm latitudes but biennial in the midwestern and northeastern states; all parts of the plant were considered medicinal. Listed in editions of the *U.S. Pharmacopoeia* from 1820 to 1910, its use led to deep and bitter feuds between botanics and regulars.

Early allopathic authors attributed lobelia's introduction into medicine to Reverend Manasseh Cutler (1742–1823) of Massachusetts who, in the *American Academy of Science* in 1785, claimed to have cured himself of asthma.[48] Several decades later, James Thacher (1754–1844), in his *American New Dispensatory*, published in 1813, attributed medical use of lobelia to the Penobscot Indians in New England. Morris Mattson in *American Vegetable Practice* (1841) likewise reported its use by the Penobscot Indians who passed it along to settlers in New England before its "discovery" by Samuel Thomson. However valid these conflicting claims might be, Thomson was using it regularly in 1805 as a remedy for colic, rheumatism, scarlet fever, erysipelas, dropsy, and other complaints in his practice, which spanned Vermont, New Hampshire, New York, and Massachusetts.[49]

The preparations of lobelia included:

1. *Infusion* (drachm to half pint of water): Used for emetic purposes, to secure full relaxation in rheumatic or convulsive situations, or for dislocations.
2. *Extract* (bruising the green herb and macerating it with diluted alcohol): Used to create a relaxing influence in febrile and acute rheumatic situations; sometimes used as a plaster for irritation of the spine.
3. *Fluid Extract* (lobelia herb macerated in alcohol and acetic acid): Used frequently as an expectorant and nauseant.
4. *Tincture* (crushed lobelia herb, including the seeds, and diluted alcohol): Used in cases of acute pleurisy, pneumonia, rheumatism, and spasmodic croup.
5. *Acetous tincture* (lobelia seeds, well ground, with distilled vinegar and diluted alcohol): Acted on the respiratory organs as a relaxant and stimulant, promoting rapid expectoration and relaxing spasms.
6. *Acetous Syiru* (acetous tincture dissolved in white sugar): Employed for same situations as acetous tincture.
7. *Oxymel, Honey of Lobelia* (tincture of bruised lobelia herb in cider vinegar and clarified honey): Used for dry and irritable coughs; less stimulating and more soothing than the acetous preparations.
8. *Oil* (pulverized seed with sulfuric ether): Given in five drop doses as an emetic.
9. *Lozenges* (acetous tincture and white sugar): A relaxing expectorant for irritable coughs.
10. *Compound Tincture of Lobelia and Capsicum, Antispasmodic Tincture, Thomson's Third Preparation* (lobelia seeds and capsicum, cypripedium, and compound tincture of myrrh): Used as powerful stimulating and relaxing compound; aroused the stomach, the circulation, and nervous system.
11. *Balsam of Honey* (tincture of lobelia, essence of anise and of sassafras, and clarified honey): Effective expectorant and antispasmodic in whooping cough and dryness of the air passages.

12. *Compound Pills* (lobelia seeds, cypripedium, asarum, and softened extract of boneset): Used as a mild nauseant and expectorant; valuable in nervousness, mild hysteria, neuralgia, nervous headache, and sleeplessness.
13. *Stomach Pill* (lobelia seeds, apocynum, hydrastis, and capsicum): Used for chronic atony of the stomach and in cases of dropsy and atonic forms of digestion.
14. *Suppositories* (lobelia seeds, simple cerate, and pulverized gum Arabic): Used for all acute pains of pelvic region and lower bowels, and especially for restlessness, chronic ovaritis, sciatica, neuralgia, and rheumatism of the womb.[50]

Regulars found it curious that both old-school Thomsonians and reformers were arrayed against the use of poisonous medicines and yet were so trustingly dependent on the lobelia plant. Throughout Thomson's career and the subsequent history of the physios, regulars recounted with predictable smugness how lobelia was a harsh, depressing drug and a powerful poison, and they were quick to publicize instances of legal suits alleging malpractice and wrongful deaths following its use.[51] Much of the initial debate had resulted from the notoriety of Thomson's own trial in 1809 before the Supreme Court in Salem, Massachusetts, for the death of Ezra Lovett, Jr., by lobelia poisoning. Thomson was acquitted, but allopths made frequent reference to the trial as proof of the drug's dangerous effects. In explaining these instances of alleged poisoning, the physios emphasized the possibility for impurities, raised questions as to whether lobelia seeds or leaves had been used, and suggested that the constitution of the patient might not have been accurately assessed before calculating the size of the dose. Negative publicity aside, lobelia remained the most important medicine in the armamentarium of botanic reformers.[52]

Germ Theory

Robert Koch's (1843–1910) description in 1876 of the life history of the anthrax bacillus elevated germ theory to a scientific basis. His discovery of the mycobacterium of tuberculosis in 1882, his identification of the cholera bacillus, and findings by scientists in subsequent years challenged many of medicine's long-held beliefs by linking a specific organism to a specific disease. Koch's postulates for the diagnosis of disease became the anchor of bacteriology and, despite the confusing use of the terms "germ," "organism," and "virus," the experimental basis upon which his evidence rested set doctors and scientists scampering to embrace the theory, adapt it to older theories, or oppose it as contrary to their particular principles of medicine.[53]

Those new treatments that developed in the wake of Koch's discovery became a matter of grave concern for the physios. Specifically, they questioned how a "deadly poison" such as the diphtheria toxin could change into a sanative agent or "antitoxin" when it was introduced into the body-laboratory of a horse. Reformers rejected the idea that serum therapy was in any way similar to the cowpox vaccine of Edward Jenner (1749–1823). Cowpox was a specific disease of the cow; when it was introduced into the human system, it removed from the human organism the food or pablum upon which the specific cowpox germ subsisted "and thus renders the field barren, so that the individual is not subject to smallpox." This was not the same as turning a "toxin" into an "antitoxin," or a diphtheric poison into a cure for diphtheria.[54]

The physio-medicalists accused regulars of pushing serum therapy "to the limit," reasoning that "in some manner, unknown at the present time, the system generates within itself certain properties, certain elements, that are antagonistic to bacteria and their toxins when the system is exposed to their action and influence." Roger T. Farley, M.D., of Chicago believed that the manufacturers and prescribers of antitoxins ignored the essential laws of nature by introducing poison into the living tissue. Although the physios did not deny the existence of bacteria or that toxins were deleterious to living tissues, they asserted that correct treatment had to account for vital force and be administered on physiological lines; any agent used to restore the integrity of the body had first to come under the influence of the vital force for tissue restoration to take place.[55]

The leaders of physio-medicine considered the so-called antitoxins as nothing less than poisonous. No amount of dilution could change their inherent virulency or convert them from a toxic to a sanative agent. Serum dilutions of diphtheria bacilli, for example, had nothing curative in their action upon the bioplasm. "So far as it goes," commented Joseph M. Thurston, "it is just as inimical and invasive to the vital integrity of the living organism as the bacillus diphtheriae and their undiluted toxins."[56] Rather than seek some form of antitoxin immunization, physios relied on capsicum and lobelia inflata to assist the vital force in asserting itself over the organs of the body and thus check the toxins in the system.[57]

In his lectures at the Physio-Medical College of Indiana, George Hasty observed that the best allopathic pathologists believed tuberculosis was dependent on a specific cause or germ (the bacillus tuberculosis) and that when the organism entered the lung tissue, it caused irritation and produced the tubercular tissue. Instead, Hasty reasoned that if tuberculosis was produced by a germ, it had to be a bioplasmic germ, not the bacillus. "It is a law of nature," he observed, "that living matter produces other living matter of the same kind, governed by the same laws and endowed with the same capabilities." In view of this fact, the allopathic theory that the bacillus was the cause of tuberculosis was false since it must of necessity produce another bacillus of the same kind. Hasty concluded that while imperfect nutrition was not the immediate cause of tuberculosis, it was nonetheless a "great cause." He agreed that tuberculosis was an infectious disease that selected constitutions already contaminated with poisonous and effluvial materials.[58]

Physios such as Thurston of Indiana came eventually to accept germ theory. Nevertheless, Thurston continued to accuse regulars of focusing their efforts on finding antiseptics to kill germs when, instead, they ought to be destroying the culture fields of germ life. He postulated the thesis that "the highest state of antisepsis is reached and maintained only through the highest grade of vital integrity and inherent resistance of the living organism." This meant destroying the conditions favorable to the growth and development of germs, or *asepsis*, rather than the killing of germs, or *antisepsis*. Eventually, he hoped that the medical profession would relegate all antitoxins and antiseptics to the dustbin of therapeutic practice.[59]

Consistent with Thurston's beliefs, physios refused to use either bichloride of mercury or carbolic acid as antiseptics, believing they did more harm than good. They preferred instead poultices of lobelia seed and elm; hayseed and wood ashes; or charcoal, hop yeast, and bayberry.

Perhaps the clearest statement of physio-medical practice came from editor George Hasty during a discussion of the use of hot water in surgical operations.

> Well, there seems to be some difference of opinion on this matter and may be all are right and may be all wrong; you may read upon this matter, and you will find that the last investigations show that the germs still remain on the instrument after being removed from the antiseptic solution, bi-chloride, etc., and hot water and soap is now the thing. Asepsis does more good than any other thing. If we can get things clean and keep them so we are doing well; alcohol will kill all germs; wash the surface to be operated on in soap and water, then apply alcohol, leaving out all poison. Dirty hands make dirty work. Some agents that are non-poisonous are just as good or better antiseptics than those that contain poison; we have seen wounds heal without even soap and water, but no harm can come from clean instruments and clean hands. The constitution of the patient may have a great deal to do with the healing of a wound; some will be bad under the best local application. A majority of cases will get well if left alone, but a larger percent will recover under good aseptic conditions. Let us use something that will not kill the living matter of the body.[60]

The physios continued in the main to be "bug cranks," believing that bacteria were "a good thing to have in a wound when they live by their own pabulum." Thurston admitted to having experimented with antiseptics but found them too strong. Instead, he reverted to the use of Thomson's Rheumatic Drops (known popularly as "No. 6"), arguing that the "best antiseptic is vital force."[61] There could never be too much emphasis on the vital energy needed to endure surgery. Excessive catharsis, or any form of depletion, would detract from the vital force in the tissue unit. Consistent with this belief, the physios practiced conservative surgery.[62]

Writing in 1894, F. O. Broady announced that it was time for physio-medicalists to take a "decided stand" on the question of bacteria since state licensing boards had begun examining applicants on the subject; this meant that bacteriology had to become a part of the curriculum and that physios needed to determine their position on whether bacteria were benign or pathogenic (i.e., disease-causing). Drawing information and criticism from among allopathic skeptics as well as from among reformers, Broady concluded that bacteria were not pathogenic; rather, disease resulted from a depressed or lowered vital action in the living organism that, in turn, caused a lowering of the standard of the organic units (meaning the secretions and excretions) and furnished a culture medium for microorganisms. Having once gained access to the living organism because of the lowered conditions of the vital fluids, microorganisms proceeded to lower the condition of the neighboring fluids and solids. But they were not in and of themselves the cause of disease.[63]

Notwithstanding the efforts of younger physios to address the question of bacteria, older practitioners were more set in their ways. M. Hermance, M.D., was not unlike many practicing reformers who, writing in 1895, continued to assert that the most rational explanation of disease causation had come from John Thomson's work on Asiatic cholera, published sixty years earlier. Thomson attributed Asiatic cholera to the "unusual destruction of animal and vegetable matter during violent and sudden changes in the weather," and the "excess of nitrous or morbid gas that was extracted by the power of heat from the decaying mass during the summer weather."[64] Hermance insisted that Thomson's theory was the most sensible ever advanced to explain the cause of cholera and was surely a fuller explanation than the microbe theory then in vogue. He concluded that Thomson's explanation applied as well to germ theory, namely, that "all the microscopical animalcule ever found in the excretions or fluids of the body in a person diseased are the result of disease, and not the cause of it."[65]

Notable exceptions aside, those physios who had been in practice for some years continued to oppose germ theory, calling Koch the "great German Bacilli-Maniac" and a "would-be scientist."[66] As one critic wrote in *Sanative Medicine*: "The bacteric hobby is at present being ridden to death and that any of us who survive for another twenty years will then laugh heartily at the fashionable craze of today, just as we now laugh at the iridectomy mania."[67] The reformers compared the search for disease specifics to the search for the philosopher's stone and, as late as 1904, their journals were still explaining how disease came first, followed by bacilli.[68] More specifically, they criticized germ theory because it lacked a working hypothesis based on the immutable laws of physiology. Until medicine returned to a more rational foundation, all of its vaunted progress and advanced methods, including bacteriology, would remain but "a splendid conglomerate of experimental concrete facts" and aimless empirical applications.[69] Most physios concurred with the comment made in 1907 by a professor at the Physio-Medical College of Indiana that "the so-called 'disease germ' is a monumental medical bugbear; it is the greatest romanticism of the age."[70]

The reformers gave deference to such terms as bacteria, tissue units, bioplasm, and other more modern terminology but continued to rely on the regimens handed down by Thomson and his disciples. This meant maintaining an "aseptic state" for the gastrointestinal tract, and using mints, balms, lobelias, vapor baths, spongings of water, and other sanative means, including electricity and magnetism, to "loosen the tissues, open the emunctories and make a way of escape to any and every deleterious matter that may exist in the system." This was the only true system based on "simplicity, truthfulness and safety."[71]

"The American"

With the celebration of individual freedom that accompanied the Jacksonian period and its aftermath, and the rejection of anything that hinted of elitism, came the repeal of medical licensing and restrictions on unlicensed practice. In effect, the claims and counterclaims of regulars, Thomsonians, homeopaths, hydropaths, eclectics, physio-medicals, and other sectarians confused legislators to the point that, rather than attempt to discern differences between and among them, they decided that the best public policy was to give citizens the right to choose their own therapeutic regimen. For both regulars and sectarians, the challenge lay in developing self-identity. Existing state and local medical societies served this purpose to some degree but, increasingly, the need arose for a broader identity. Regulars saw in organization the means for defending their educational distinctiveness; a weapon in the fight for protective legislation; and a symbol for a uniform physiology and pathology as taught in the best schools in Europe and America. For sectarians, organization served similar purposes. They wanted it for reasons of self-promotion, self-defense (equal rights under the law), and a desire to expand their regional platforms. For both, the most significant outcome of these efforts was the transformation of their voluntary associations into national organizations. Allopathy accomplished this by calling for a national convention in New York in 1846. The first meeting proved to be little more than a gathering of New York physicians, but the 1847 convention in Philadelphia included 250 representatives from twenty-one states. By the close of the third meeting in Baltimore in 1848, the American Medical Association had become a national organization.[1]

Tribulations

The first effort to organize botanic physicians occurred fourteen years before the founding of the American Medical Association, when Samuel Thomson called for delegates from the Friendly Botanic Societies to convene in Columbus, Ohio, in 1832. The convention, composed of delegates from each state, used the opportunity to prepare a constitution and bylaws, to share information on plant remedies but, more importantly, to discuss means to combat state legislation limiting their practice. By 1835, Alva Curtis and other botanics, hoping to build a more lasting legacy through the establishment of medical colleges and infirmaries, had begun to challenge Thomson's leadership. Schism between Thomson and the supporters of Curtis became a reality in 1838 when Curtis withdrew from the U.S. Thomsonian Convention to form the Independent Thomsonian Botanic Society; Thomson, in turn, organized the U.S. Thomsonian Society. State botanic societies responded to the schism by announcing their allegiance to one or the other and a few chose not to affiliate at all. Subsequent meetings of the U.S. Thomsonian Society proved disappointing as it became clear that old-guard Thomsonism could no longer denigrate formal medical education. For every advocate of old-guard Thomsonism there were two or more critics anxious to realize the full potential of botanic medicine. As the editor of the *Western Medical Reformer* explained in 1837,

> Every enlightened friend to the Botanic practice must deplore the presumption of ignorant men, who imagine that by purchasing a Thomsonian book, and reading over a mass of heterogenous nonsense, the sum total of Botanic medical practice is obtained. The man who gives up his agricultural or mechanical pursuit, to acquire a livelihood as a botanic practitioner, may be vain enough

to think he has been transformed into a worker of miracles; but common sense should admonish the afflicted to guard against the general herd of Thomsonians, as much as against the prodigal practice of calomel and the lancet. To be a judicious and successful practitioner of the Botanic School, we contend that a radical knowledge of the vegetable kingdom is essentially necessary to give a claim to public confidence in the reformed practice of medicine. The miraculous power of transforming farmers and mechanics into doctors in a moment, is doubted in the present day.[2]

The cause of botanic medicine had also been weakened by sectional differences, petty jealousies, and doctrinal disagreements. Not surprisingly, the consensus among reformers to establish medical colleges broke down when it came to determining the nature and extent of botanic reform. Complicating matters further, the reformers were undecided on the half dozen names that circulated among the schismatics. Furthermore, eclectics had managed to steal credit for the petitions the reformers had organized in the 1840s against New York's medical laws and, claiming to be the only true agents of change, succeeded in capturing leadership positions in many state botanic societies. Of course, defenders of reform medicine found it difficult to accept the fact that their colleagues could have been drawn into the eclectic camp except through deceit. "Numbers of our good men were drawn into [the eclectic school] unawares," complained William H. Cook of Cincinnati, "and unwillingly were giving their support to this diluted form of allopathy."[3]

In the context of these events Curtis and the reform wing of the Thomsonians met in Baltimore in 1852. Botanic reformers from four southeastern states issued an invitation to bring all true reformers into an affiliation built around certain agreed-upon principles. Professor J. Thomas Coxe of Georgia urged that each state send five delegates, a plan designed to prevent any one state or region of the country from dominating the convention. Ultimately, ten states sent delegates to the meeting— Connecticut, Delaware, Georgia, Maryland, Massachusetts, New York, Ohio, Pennsylvania, South Carolina, and Virginia.[4]

Curtis and his reform wing of independent Thomsonians dominated the convention and used their influence to organize the delegates into the Reformed Medical Association of the United States with himself as president. He also worked with a committee consisting of professors

L. Bankston and J. Thomas Coxe of the Southern Botanico-Medical College at Macon, Georgia; Isaac Miller Comings of the Metropolitan Medical College of New York City; William F. Smith of Philadelphia; H. F. Johnson of Massachusetts; S. L. Swormstedt of Maryland; and Samuel J. Watson of Virginia to develop a platform of principles to represent the beliefs of the association:

Resolved, By the Reformed Medical Association of the United States that medical science, pertaining altogether to natural subjects, must be in itself as fixed and definite as any other natural science.

Resolved, That the reason why medical men have not learned it, is they have attempted to base it upon the violation of physical laws, which are ever variable, instead of those laws themselves, which are immutable: they have built their systems on what they call pathology—or rather they have pronounced that pathology which is only deranged physiology, and built upon error.

Resolved, That the reformers of past times have failed to perfect their practice, because of the impossibility of doing it while they retain the false notion that the science is based on pathology, or the doctrine that physiological derangements are disease.

Resolved, That the fundamental principles of true medical science are not pathological but physiological.

Resolved, That disease is not vital action deranged or obstructed, increased or diminished, but any condition of the organs in which they are unable to perform their natural functions: a condition that permanently deranges, obstructs, or diminishes vital action, and in this sense is a unit.

Resolved, That irritation, fever, inflammation—terms used to signify increased, deranged, obstructed, or accumulated vital action in the nervous or vascular systems—are not disease, but physiological symptoms of disease; and are not to be directly subdued, but always to be aided in their ultimate design and intention in removing obstructions and restoring the nervous and circulatory equilibrium.

Resolved, That suppuration is to be encouraged and promoted whenever there is accumulated morbific matter to be removed; that gangrene, being no part of inflammation, but a purely chemical process in opposition to all vital action, and occurring only when vital action has wholly ceased, the associating of it with inflammation, and treating the latter as tending to terminate in the former, has been a source of immense mischief in medication.

Resolved, That it is the duty of the practitioner to reject in toto every means and process, which, in its nature and tendency, in authorized medicinal quantities, degrees, or modes of application, has been known to have directly destroyed human life, or permanently injured the tissue, or deranged the physiological action, and to use those, and those only, which have a direct tendency to aid the vital organs in the removal of causes of disease and the restoration of health and vigor.

Resolved, That the agents of this character are not confined to the vegetable kingdom, but are found in every department of nature, and to be "seized upon wherever found."

Resolved, That though we shall exercise charity towards the ignorance and prejudices of all men, we can count no one a true medical reformer who rejects the doctrines of the foregoing resolutions.[5]

Previous to the drafting of these principles, there had been considerable sympathy but little uniformity of thought among the independent Thomsonians. Beyond the narrow border of Thomson's principles, each had been left to his own idiosyncratic devices. Not surprisingly, the platform proved difficult to draft since the areas of medical agreement were as varied as the regional differences of those in attendance. Both a constitution and platform of principles were presented to the association membership but the diversity of opinion among the participants resulted in only a portion being ratified. A year later, the western reformers (Curtis supporters) met in Cincinnati and adopted the principles as framed in Baltimore the previous year. Those who attended the convention and who represented the more liberal wing of reform Thomsonism (some of whom openly sided with the eclectics) refused to agree with the principles and their rancor was such that the association never met again.[6]

Before the Reformed Medical Association of the United States became defunct, its leaders called for reformers to support their fledgling schools and medical journals; urge the adoption of reform pharmacy; encourage regularized fees; and assign to the Metropolitan Medical College of New York City the task of publishing a United States reformed medical dispensatory. None of these objectives was realized, and subsequent efforts undertaken in 1857, 1859, and 1877 to organize another national meeting also failed. Looking back on the 1852 Baltimore convention, William H. Cook recalled that while it had begun with many good intentions, it had made mistakes, including the attempt to legislate for those reformers not represented at the meeting. As a result, it failed to materialize as an incorporated organization.[7] In the interim, the eastern reformers representing Pennsylvania, Delaware, New Jersey, Maryland, and Virginia founded the Middle States Reformed Medical Society; and the southern states, represented by Alabama, Arkansas, Kentucky, Mississippi, Tennessee, and Virginia (which joined both) formed the Southern Reform Medical Association.[8]

In 1879, the Ohio Physio-Medical Society called for a national convention to be held in 1881. Some state societies responded positively to the proposition; others ignored the invitation altogether. In states that lacked organized societies, individual physicians had no formal association through which to express any official support. The Ohio society, concerned that only true physio-medicalists be involved, insisted that the convention be constituted of "properly chosen representatives, apportioned on some plan that might be devised by the committees of the different States." This, wrote editor William H. Cook in the *Cincinnati Medical Gazette and Recorder,* would eliminate diploma merchants, eclectics, nostrum vendors, and abortionists from gaining admittance. States without an organized society could still participate provided that physios practicing in those states appointed a committee to represent their interests. In so doing, each state would be guaranteed proportionate representation without any one state controlling the convention.[9] As a followup to the association's request, Cook and H. E. Hoke submitted a proposal for an assemblage based on the following points: An equable representation among the states; strict adherence to physio-medical principles; and membership restricted to graduates of colleges giving "a full course of instruction by an organized corps of teachers."[10] The two doctors feared that if the terms for membership were left to a mass meeting, a simple majority could "fix" the qualifications and thereby admit "disreputable persons" into the association.[11] These persons, warned Hoke, "are always anxious to use [associations] to float themselves into professional standing." Both he and Cook intended to prevent this from happening.[12]

In contrast to the Ohio plan, the Indiana physios proposed a convention of *all* reformers regardless of their membership in a state organization; once convened, the attendees of the convention would establish a permanent association and fix the qualifications for membership. Fearing that the Ohio physios might try to dominate the convention, S. M. White, M.D., of the Physio-Medical College of Indiana proposed that no professor could hold a position as officer in the convention. White and the Indiana physios were troubled by Cook's public stand against Alva Curtis and preferred not to have the convention used to spotlight their feud. Specifically, the Indiana physios did not want the convention to become a battleground for determining which diplomas should or should not be recognized.[13]

Cook felt that if the convention admitted all who applied, "It would be a serious question whether physio-medicalism has an actual existence, or whether it is but a whimsical appendage to eclecticism." Specifically, individuals who had bought their diplomas from Curtis, John Buchanan, William Paine, and others in the name of physio-medicalism would be equal with those who held their credentials by honest means. This Cook refused to allow. Standing his ground, he affirmed that while he had no personal interest in seeking office in any new organization, he found it difficult to believe that professors in physio-medical colleges should be denied the rights of other members. "It seems to me," he wrote White, "that this would be discriminating . . . against the most effective, hardworking, self-sacrificing men in our ranks."[14] He insisted that any convention in which the Ohio reformers participated would have to be formed on the basis of an equitable system of representation, meaning that only states with an organized society would have an official voice. Otherwise, the state where the convention was held could "rush in its convenient men" and control policy issues that were national in scope.[15]

Troubled by the manner in which the Indiana physios were attempting to control the convention, Cook decided to publish the correspondence between himself and White. In their letters, none of which were very friendly, Cook accused the Indiana physios of vacillating on the issue of credentialing; showing a willingness to accept disreputable physicians as equals in a mass convention; and not adhering to the true strictures of physio-medicalism. Uncompromising, he demanded that any call for a national convention declare unequivocally that the delegates be true to their practice; that the authority of the convention derive from the delegates who came from states with organized official associations; that no state having sent delegates would be deprived of proportional representation; and that no state which stood aloof from organizing state societies could expect to have the same advantages as those who sent delegates.[16] Under no circumstances, Cook vowed, would Ohio submit to a sham convention since it would simply reduce the role of delegates from other states by making them become the "tails to help Indiana fly her kite."[17] Recalling an earlier time and an earlier battle, he remarked that Indiana "shall not be the State to attempt to break down a National Convention she cannot control, as she did in 1852."[18] Nevertheless, with Indiana's refusal to agree to the Ohio proposition, the convention failed to materialize.

Indiana was not alone it its obstinacy. According to A. H. Baird, M.D., of Jackson, Michigan, most physios agreed on the need for a national convention but felt that the Ohio physios were preaching nationalism while practicing sectionalism; delegates from states without associations had just as much right to attend a national convention as states with established organizations. Let all true physio-medicalists be invited to meet in convention, he argued, and then let the convention decide by vote who shall and who shall not be members, and make rules and regulations for future meetings. After a specified number of years, the convention could then choose to be composed only of delegates from different state associations. At that time, physio-medicalists in states lacking established associations would be prohibited from having a vote except by consent of the convention.[19]

The matter of a national convention remained unresolved until March 1883, when George Hasty of the Physio-Medical College of Indiana called for a meeting in May of that year—barely two months away. Cook cried foul, claiming that the notice was too short. He also accused Hasty of being the principal impediment to the earlier organizing efforts in 1879 and 1880. While Cook added that he would be glad to meet at Indianapolis or anywhere else under the banner of true physiomedicalism, he adamantly refused to be a party to "selling out this cause to corrupt men—men whose standing is well known to us, some of whom deserve to be in the penitentiary and whom we shall not hesitate to point out if we find it necessary." By inference, Cook expressed a feeling shared by other reformers that physio-medicalism had become an umbrella for a variety of dubious medical and licensing frauds whose notoriety had eroded the integrity of the sect.[20]

Hasty published Cook's comments in the *Physio-Medical Journal,* accusing the Ohio reformer of having devised every means possible to exclude bonafide colleagues from the convention, and using representation as a ruse to control the national association. In reality, Hasty pointed out, Cook was carrying on a personal vendetta to exclude friends of his rival Alva Curtis. Hasty referred to Cook as "pious William," having a "vengeful disposition" against the Indiana physios and the true followers of Curtis.[21] Believing that further delay was "suicidal" and that, for thirty years, the cause of physio-medicalism had been without a "guiding head," Hasty called for reformers to meet in Indianapolis and to finally organize a national association.[22]

In May 1883, forty-eight physios (including three women) representing nine states met at Indianapolis and organized the American Association of Physio-Medical Physicians and Surgeons. Of this number, twenty-four delegates came from Indiana, eleven from Ohio, five from Illinois, two each from Iowa and New York, and one each from California, Minnesota, Nebraska, and Texas.[23] The delegates elected A. F. Elliot, M.D., of Minneapolis as chairman and Melville C. Keith, M.D., of Nebraska, as secretary. Cook made his presence immediately known by proclaiming that no diploma buyer, diploma seller, or abortionist should take part in the meeting. He also demanded that only those who practiced without using poisons and who likwise opposed fraudulent diplomas should be accepted into the organization. Having made his "pious" statements to an indulging audience, Cook felt appeased on those issues that had rankled him since 1879.[24]

The convention proceeded to appoint a Committee on Constitution and Platform of Principles and then recessed to await the committee's report. Two hours later, the committee reported to the convention its platform of principles.

Section 1. The Science of Medicine, like all other sciences is based upon the laws of nature, and Medical Art can be true and reliant only when it is in harmony with these laws.

Sec. 2. Disease is that condition of bodily structures in which they are unable to perform their functions in a natural manner, which condition disturbs the harmony and equilibrium of the system; and the object of medical science is the restoration of diseased structures to their natural state as far as possible, that they may be enabled again to perform their office.

Sec. 3. Physiological actions are always resistive to the causes of disease, and tend to the restoration of health when this is disturbed; and remedial treatment should harmonize with physiological efforts, conserving and assisting the inherent curative powers of the system.

Sec. 4. Observing this physiological standard as the only true guide in the Curative Art, no article should be used in the cure of disease that by its nature tends to damage the integrity of structures or impairs the vitality of tissues; hence, all measures that are injurious and all agents that are poisonous are to be rejected from medical practice as being in themselves causes of disease and not promoters of health.[25]

The convention also approved a constitution that formally established the American Association of Physio-Medical Physicians and Surgeons (known by members as "The American") whose members were required to conform to the sentiments of its platform. In a demonstrable show of unity, Cook nominated George Hasty for president, and Jacob Redding nominated A. F. Elliot of Minnesota. Hasty was unanimously elected president, with Elliot as first vice-president, William F. Tait of Illinois as second vice-president, William Wesley Cook of Ohio as secretary, and John A. Morehouse of Indiana as treasurer.[26] When the convention ended, the physios were pleased with the harmonious achievement of their objective and looked forward to the 1884 meeting in Cincinnati. In describing the meeting, William H. Cook observed that "perhaps no medical assemblage ever accomplished so much in so little time." He applauded the unanimity of sentiment and expressed his personal pleasure that would-be "disturbing elements" had wisely chosen to stay away from the convention.[27] In the meantime, Hasty urged the members to recruit other physios into the association, collect statistics noting improvements in their methods of practice, and bring to the next convention a feeling of common good.[28]

The following year, the association convened at Greenwood Hall in Cincinnati and was called to order by president George Hasty. William H. Cook welcomed the convention to the Queen City and to the "fountain-head of Physio-Medicalism," sparred with Melville C. Keith regarding the credentials of one of the members and then surprised the assembly by announcing a resolution to change the name of the society to the American Physio-Medical Association.[29]

This was followed by a discussion of papers on theory and practice during which time Cook and other delegates hotly debated the germ theory of diphtheria. Most of the discussants refused to believe in the germ theory of causation, preferring to hold first to local causation, then constitutional. Melville C. Keith, author of *Diphtheria: History, Causes, Symptoms, Prevention and Cure* (1879), argued that diphtheria was a constitutional disease arising from excesses of starchy food. Believing that the regular school of medicine had ignored the plants, herbs, and flowers that were the bases of true medicine, he recommended a treatment consisting of wildcherry root, culver's root, pleurisy root, prickly ash berries, and rhubarb.[30]

Cook was equally critical of the theory, having noticed that no germs were found in the blood current, but merely in local blood that oozed from capillaries in the decaying parts. Germs had nothing to do with the cause of disease and existed only because disease had damaged the tissues and the germs there "find a place to exist, like maggots in bad meat." The danger of the theory was that it encouraged physicians to unwittingly become "poisoners" in order to destroy the germ. The whole idea was little more than "wild speculation," which he was convinced would soon be thrown aside.[31]

The second day of the convention began like the first, with Cook and Thurston again sparring in the section on theory and practice and with

Thurston asking why Cook felt so "afraid of investigation." Cook responded that he had no desire to limit the investigative side of medicine; rather, he wished there was less theoretical and more "practical discussion" of the doctrine of vitality on which physio-medicalism was founded. No doubt Cook intended to chastise Thurston and his colleagues at the Indiana college for their lengthy philosophical discourses on vitalism in the *Physio-Medical Journal*.[32]

On the afternoon of the second day, tempers flared as the convention turned to the issue of where to hold the 1885 meeting. C. T. Bedford of Indiana invited the association to meet once again in Indianapolis, while W. F. Tait suggested Galesburg, Illinois. Melville C. Keith objected to Illinois, arguing that he "had lived there and left," and besides, he objected to holding a meeting where an allopathic state board of health controlled the examination and licensing of physicians. Cook supported the Galesburg location, noting that returning so soon to Indianapolis would demonstrate to the world that the association was regional and not national. After more than an hour of debate, the vote was tied, whereupon the president (from Indiana) decided in favor of Indianapolis.[33]

In order to appease those who had opposed the convention site, the delegates elected William H. Cook as the convention's next president; A. F. Elliot as first vice-president; O. W. F. Snyder as second vice-president; and D. H. Stafford of Indiana as treasurer. Both J. R. Smith of Missouri and A. W. Fisher of Indiana were nominated for secretary. Cook rose to support Smith's nomination but was declared out of order. Behind the disagreement lay a substantial issue, namely, whether Fisher, who was not one of the bonafide delegates of the Indiana physio-medical association, could hold office. In the convention vote, the Indiana faction mustered support sufficient to elect Fisher as secretary.[34] By this time, relations between and among the delegates had deteriorated to such an abysmal level that when William Wesley Cook rose to read friendly greetings to the delegates from reformers in Illinois, Texas, California, and Michigan who had been unable to attend, the convention promptly declared him out of order.[35]

In reflecting on their second annual meeting, George Hasty recalled that much work had been left unfinished due to personal jealousies and professional rivalries. One thing was certain; when any one physio (meaning William H. Cook) set himself up as the "oracle" of physio-medicalism "to whom all must bow," and who attempted to "pocket" the association, such efforts would be quickly discovered and put down. The same held true of those who attempted to "stuff the ballot box" or pursue a "gunning expedition" against one of the members. Lastly, he attacked the secretary's (William Wesley Cook of Cincinnati) official report of the meeting as "largely a bundle of official perverseness."[36]

In the months prior to the 1885 meeting, Cook accused the national organization of being in league with elements that had failed to serve the best interests of botanical medicine. Reputedly there had been representatives from nine states at the first meeting, but in truth, he pointed out, only seven states were represented since some attendees had improperly identified themselves where they had once lived, not where they now resided. Cook also took exception to those physios who stood aloof from the organization while they insisted on representation. It was just such an attitude that had left the physio-medicals without representation on state examining and licensing boards. As long as botanic reformers failed to attend to their interests, they left the field to allopathy and other sectarian groups to secure the most advantageous laws for themselves and their societies. "If we want an equal voice in such laws," he wrote in the *Cincinnati Medical Gazette and Recorder*, "we also must organize societies and enter upon hard work."[37]

The third annual session of the American met at Indianapolis in May 1885 and was immediately consumed in controversy. Hasty opened the meeting by calling the association's attention to the "gross errors" in the secretary's report of the 1884 meeting. It was "a miserably garbled affair . . . utterly unworthy a place of the records and incapable of correction except by purging the whole thing."[38] Matters deteriorated further when acting president A. F. Elliot of Minneapolis announced he had received a letter from president-elect William H. Cook resigning his office and his membership in the association. In his letter, Cook also reported the resignations of second vice-president O. W. F. Snyder; chair of the board of censors W. F. Tait; members William Wesley Cook and J. A. Morehouse of the board of censors; chair of gynecology H. E. Hoke; chair of obstetrics J. R. Smith; and individual representatives from Illinois, Indiana, Ohio, Missouri, California, Kentucky, and Nebraska.[39] As Cook explained, the resignations stemmed from the association's "open advocacy" of doctrines opposed to physio-medicalism; its initiation of discussions with "eclecto-allopathic" representatives; the fact that some members had publicly advertised themselves as eclectics; that first vice-president A. F. Elliot had become a member and officer in the Eclectic Society of Minnesota; and that "narrow sectional prejudices" had been manifested by prominent members of the association. These facts convinced Cook that the association represented physio-medicalism in name only. In reality, it was "an electo-allopathic society, sectional in character, and damaging to the cause of true physio-medicalism."[40]

Unperturbed by the exodus, George Hasty announced to the assembled delegates that the resignation of these malcontents had not injured the inner strength of the association. He then filled their vacancies on the various boards and committees and, through the association's committee on committees, proposed a resolution denouncing the charges made by the former members.[41] The resolution denied as spurious the claims that the association had become eclectic or eclecto-allopathic. Until the secessionists appeared before the society with the proper proofs of the charges they made, the association branded their accusations false and malicious, sullying the fair name of the organization and its membership. The remaining association members adopted the resolution unanimously.[42]

With the malcontents gone, subsequent sessions of the American lacked the dissension that dominated the first three years of its existence. Reminiscent of Thomson's earlier friendly societies, the meetings focused on the interchange of ideas, views, prescriptions, and inquiries among physicians. Because the meetings were small, the reformers sat as a committee of the whole to discuss specific case histories, with doctors giving advice on their favorite remedies. Often, they focused on single topics such as spermatorrhea, colic, or consumption. Meetings were unstructured, with the president of the association acting as discussion leader.[43]

The twenty-first annual session met in Indianapolis in 1903 and adopted new bylaws; designated the *Physio-Medical Record* as the official organ of the association; urged the collection of statistics on physio-medical practice; encouraged the investigation of certain diseases and proposed cures; and campaigned for the organization of state associations where none existed. Finally, the association urged the preparation of an official history of the physio-medical system of medicine.[44]

Two years later, at the 1905 meeting in Indianapolis, Joseph M. Thurston again urged better use of statistics. "As you know," he chided, "we claim to be able to treat disease with more success than the physicians of other schools of medicine do. They tell us to produce our records, but we have none to produce."[45] The same was true of medical research. A.W. Titse encouraged his fellow reformers to learn what the microscope could teach. "We as physio-medicalists should not fall into such error as to let the facts and principles of physio-medicalism work for themselves and wait and pray that sometimes they might prevail." There was no longer any excuse to avoid research and investigation. Unfortunately for both Titse and Thurston, only seventy-five physios were present at the meeting to hear their concerns.[46]

The lack of statistical evidence to substantiate the superiority of their medical system had been an issue as well as a personal crusade for Thurston. "As to the physio-medical plan of treatment of cholera, and its superiority over the other schools," he observed, "I am sorry to say I have nothing to offer either from statistics, or personal experience; for, here, as in all other forms of disease, we feel that dire want of . . . clinical statistics."[47] Thurston advocated preparing and retaining complete case-books on patients. Not until reformers could demonstrate through clinical statistics the results of sanative medication could they remove the discrimination they faced in access to public hospitals. The demand for equal rights required the statistical demonstration that reform medicine truly worked.[48]

In December 1906, a group of physios, no doubt troubled by their dwindling numbers, gathered at the home of William Paul Brickley to establish the first annual meeting of the Association of Pioneer Physio-Medicalists. The association was supposedly national in scope, open to all physios who had been members of the profession for at least twenty-five years. Actually, all of the charter members were from Indiana: James A. Stafford of Millville; Willard Paul Brickley and Jacob Redding of Anderson; C.T. Bedford of Indianapolis; and Joseph M. Thurston of Richmond. Not unlike the American, this new association of pioneer physios continued to reflect the Indiana influence on botanic reform.[49]

The association dedicated itself to recording the experiences of the sect's earliest members. To achieve this, the members promised to preserve the principles, practices, and scientific traditions of physio-medicalism; record the biographies, notable facts, and professional experience of pioneer practitioners; gather facts and records pertaining to drug formulas, prescriptions, and practices of individual doctors; collect interesting personal articles such as books belonging to the pioneer founders of physio-medicalism; advise the younger generation of physios on the need for "harmonizing of modern didactic and laboratory methods with the fundamental principles required by sanative medicine"; aid in the financial endowment of the departments of the college; counsel with both physios and physio-medical colleges on the "effect, condition, and improvement of our laws in their bearings upon medical education and practice"; and promulgate through literature and lectures the truths of sanative medicine.[50]

The association's objectives were partially realized when a few articles highlighting their history began to appear in the pages of the *Physio-Medical Record;* but the avenues for publication declined dramatically by 1906. With so few young men and women choosing botanic medicine, with endowment monies barely evident, and with the emerging power of the American Medical Association and state licensing boards, the reformers found themselves ill prepared to face the future, let alone look reflectively on their past.

Medical Examining Boards

In many states, homeopaths and eclectics had succeeded in establishing their own medical examining boards, or they had secured representation with regulars on composite boards. The physios, on the other hand, suffered along with the hydropaths, osteopaths, and other fringe sects by failing oftentimes to secure similar representation. Because of their absence on these boards, the physios were often forced to seek licenses through eclectic or homeopathic boards or through those same representatives on composite boards.[51] Recognizing that regulars controlled the majority of board appointments and that their relationship with eclectics and homeopaths was not always good, the physios knew only too well that few of their graduates would survive a vote. "Of all the underhanded schemes that have ever been concocted by the regulars to down the irregulars, this is perhaps the most contemptible," commented E. Bufkin, M.D., in the *Physio-Medical Journal* in 1893. Only if all schools, including physio-medicalist, were included on these boards, and in sufficient numbers, would the legislation stand the test of fairness. He concluded that the purpose of the legislation was not to ensure fairness but to provide a legal method to prevent irregulars from practicing medicine.[52]

The eclectics did not welcome either the criticisms of the physios or, for that matter, their masquerading as nominal eclectics for purposes of licensing. Their air of ignorance and "windy bombast," remarked H. L. Webster, M.D., editor of the *California Medical Journal* (eclectic), disgraced many educated eclectics. "We will not assert that physio-medicalists are all ignorant, or that eclectics are all wise," he wrote, "but we do assert that the teaching in physio colleges has as a rule been very superficial, except so far as the management of disease is concerned."[53] Webster accused physio-medicalism of neglecting anatomy, physiology, and pathology, and taking a "peculiar and melancholy step into the past." Its followers had become "Ishmaelites whose hands have been against every medical man, and against whom the whole medical world has been almost obliged to close its doors on account of its abusive tendencies and obstreperous assaults." Webster opined that much of the criticism directed at eclectics had resulted from the public's inability to distinguish eclectics from other reform groups.[54]

Because of this reputed confusion, eclectic boards of medical examiners, beginning in 1888 in California, refused to issue licenses to holders of physio-medical diplomas, arguing that they had used the eclectic boards to pass through "the portal of legal entry into the medical profession of the state"; but they were too parsimonious to participate in eclectic medical societies, pay their annual dues, or even establish societies of their own.[55] The physios responded with predictable rancor, protesting that the board was ignorant of the curriculum of physio-medical institutions. More disheartening for the physios was the fact that, with the exception of the Medical Society of the State of California (regular), the Eclectic Medical Society of the State of California, and the California State Homeopathic Medical Society, no other state organization existed in California to examine applications for certificates and examinations. This meant that, without a sponsor, the physios could not legally practice in California. To the extent that the eclectics and homeopaths chose this course of action in other states meant fewer and fewer avenues for physios to enter into licensed practice.[56]

As a general principle, the physios considered examining and licensing boards as un-American. A. A. Abernathy, M.D., of Morristown,

Indiana, categorized them as a European custom designed by old-school doctors to destroy alternative medical systems. The truth was, he wrote, the AMA wanted to break down every system of medicine except allopathy. Abernathy thought each state should regulate medical colleges by requiring that they teach certain branches of science "necessary to the intelligent practice of medicine and surgery. Then, if a faculty wants to teach a *pathy,* let them teach it and use it to their hearts' content. If another wants to teach an *ism,* let them do it, and let none dare molest or make them afraid."[57] If students took a curriculum common to *all* schools, passed the courses and received a diploma, they should be entitled to all the rights, honors, and privileges pertaining to the medical profession. Similarly, George Hasty wrote: "Let the diploma from an honorable medical college, giving a full course of instructions be the license to practice medicine." Anything else was unfair. "Physio-medicalists are willing to let 'regularism' weed its own garden," he reasoned. "But it has no business to go into its neighbor's potato patch to cull, until it knows something about its neighbor's business."[58]

In Washington state, the regulars worked hard for the so-called Power's Bill that created a board of nine examiners, two of whom were homeopaths. Governor Elisha P. Ferry vetoed the bill; a substitute Eddy Bill then passed, leaving the matter of appointment entirely with the governor. The regulars urged the governor to appoint only those of the "old school"; when he refused, he was condemned in unmeasured terms. In an effort to achieve better balance, Ferry appointed a mixed board with a homeopath as president, a regular as secretary, and a physio as treasurer. The physios applauded Ferry's stand but privately lamented the composite board as "humbug."[59]

If the regulars were truly honest with themselves, argued Joseph M. Thurston, they would recognize there were many different but equally legitimate theories of disease causation. Therefore, legislation mandating boards of examination and registration constructed of old-school members, or even of mixed representatives, ignored the reality of osteopathy, homeopathy, hydropathy, and other legally chartered sects that practiced outside orthodoxy. Ideally, every individual who applied for licensure should be required to pass a rigid examination under the censorship of a board "made only by the members of the school or sect to which the applicant professes to adhere and practice." Alternatively, there should be equality across the different systems of medicine. This meant an equal number of members from each school on every composite board.[60]

Siren Appeals

In 1891, a Baltimore physician, in the journal *Medical Age*, called for the establishment of a society to encourage cooperation across the different systems of medicine. The organization, to be known as the National Progressive Medical Practitioners Union, would urge the passage of legislation to ensure that a license to practice in one state would be valid in every other state. The organization would unite irregular, reform, and progressive physicians into a political action group that demanded equal treatment before the law. This meant that physio-medicalists, homeopaths, and eclectics, or any other qualified irregulars, would have the same rights and privileges to practice medicine as allopaths, as long as they possessed a legal diploma from a chartered medical college in the United States. Holding that no one branch or school of medicine could learn all there was to know, that the various schools of therapeutic theory created healthy competition, and that competition "creates study and energy from which comes progress," it was hoped the union would advocate an end to the monopoly of regulars over the practice of medicine. Physios supported the proposed union, but no evidence exists that it ever materialized. No doubt the same factors that kept the sectarians divided among themselves continued to detract from efforts to minimize their differences.[61]

Other efforts were only marginally successful. In October 1894, physicians meeting in Indianapolis formed the American Association of Physicians and Surgeons as nondenominational, inviting into its membership the advocates of regular medicine, homeopathy, eclecticism, physio-medicalism, hygienic medicine, hydrotherapeutics, and electrotherapeutics. Initially its members came principally from Indiana, but later membership indicated a broader participation. At the first annual meeting in January 1895, in Indianapolis, members elected Dr. C. Edison Covey of Michigan as president and Dr. Russell C. Kelsey of Indianapolis as secretary; vice-presidents were elected from each of the states

represented in the association. The 1896 meeting also met in Indianapolis, followed by a 1897 meeting in Buffalo.

Organized under the auspices of this association was the American
Medical College of Indianapolis, with a faculty of thirty professors. Out
of respect for all schools, students could choose regular, homeopathic,
eclectic, or physio-medical courses from the curriculum. This innova-
tive idea, however altruistic, fell on deaf ears. Eclectic John M. Scudder
condemned the college and the association for having succeeded in
gathering into its fold "the queer of all schools." Seen as a pariah by all
medical groups and their associations, the school failed to sustain support. Its first class graduated in 1895 and its last class graduated barely a
year later; the college closed in 1897.[62]

The Jeremiahs among the physios continued to warn members
that, without organization, their future remained in jeopardy. Those who
failed to organize would be at the mercy of other sects and state legislatures. "If you don't take care of yourselves, nobody will take care of you,"
warned the editor of the *Physio-Medical Journal* in 1890. "Rest assured
that the effort to legislate is not dead by any means, and to depend upon
other sects to grant certificates is very bad nonsense. The thing has been
tried. The liberality of sects in medicine in that respect has all eked out.
Organize. Have committees to see to the legislation question. Demand
justice. Don't lie dormant until you are tied hand and foot, but put yourselves in battle array."[63]

At their meetings, physios complained frequently that certain colleagues acted as though they were ashamed of being classified as physio-
medicalists. Many, in fact, tried to pass as eclectics, homeopaths, and
even regulars. They seemed embarrassed by their origins even though
they accused regulars of having borrowed many of their own medicines.
One physio, who admitted to the unpopularity of the school, remarked
that on those occasions when he had been mistaken for a homeopath,
he made no effort to correct the error.[64]

When the American Medical Association reorganized at the turn of
the century, included in its plan was a re-examination of the 1847 code of
ethics that had prohibited consultation with sectarians. The new code,
approved in 1903, recommended the broadest dictates of humanity be
used in meeting the challenge of disease and medical emergencies. To
achieve this objective, the document authorized state and local medical

societies to admit into their fellowship all legally recognized physicians, provided they no longer advertised themselves as sectarians.

The American Association of Physio-Medical Physicians and Surgeons warned its members to weigh carefully the propriety of joining local branches of the American Medical Association. Admittedly, regulars had been involved in "earnest, honest research work," but they had insisted on "political exclusiveness." They had, for example, acquired full control over the army and navy medical departments where 4,308 physicians held salaried appointments. Not a single one of those appointees adhered publicly to a sectarian school. Arguing that sectarianism was inconsistent with medical science since there was but one science of medicine, regulars had convinced government officials that there should be but one school of medical practice.[65] Notwithstanding these protests, many physios used licensing boards to pass as eclectics and homeopaths; and these same individuals, when given the opportunity, used the invitation of the American Medical Association to mainstream into regular medicine.

An Empty Sack

By the 1880s, most local and state physio-medical associations had died for lack of members. The editor of the *Physio-Medical Journal* reported in 1880 that the Iowa, Kansas, Michigan, Missouri, New York, Ohio, Pennsylvania, and Texas physios had failed to provide updated information on their activities, and he presumed their societies were defunct.[66] On occasion, the fears proved false as when, in 1907, the Oklahoma Physio-Medical Association of Physicians and Surgeons organized.[67] However, the belated birth of the Oklahoma association had less to do with ordinary association activities than with the requirement of the Oklahoma state board that out-of-state applicants for reciprocity secure the endorsement of their respective state societies. Without an official association, out-of-state physios could not practice in Oklahoma.[68]

Physio-medicalism was strongest in Ohio, Indiana, Illinois, and Iowa, with additional followings in Texas, Oregon, and Washington. At its peak, probably fewer than 2,500 were practicing physio-medicalism at any one time. Even this number is probably inflated since the national organization, formed in 1883, claimed only 150 members. According to a survey in 1894, regulars numbered 72,028; eclectics, 10,292; homeopaths, 9,648; and physios, 1,553.[69] On average, physio-medical colleges graduated 21.6 physicians annually between 1881 and 1890. Of the state societies, Indiana was the oldest, having organized in 1863; others existed in Ohio, Illinois, Iowa, Michigan, and Washington.[70] In 1900, the Ohio Medical Directory listed 1,162 sectarians, nearly 19 percent of all physicians; of that number, 769 were homeopaths, 342 were eclectics, 41 were physio-medicalists, and 7 were minor cultists. By 1905, the percentage of sectarians had declined to 17 percent, and by 1917, they represented only 13 percent of the practicing physicians in the state.[71]

Unlike the American Medical Association which, by the turn of the twentieth century, was fast building a strong national organization on the shoulders of even stronger state and local associations, the physios found themselves depending on a national organization that was little more than an empty shell for lack of local and state chapters. In an age when the determinants of power rested on the strength of local and state societies, the future of physio-medicalism lay ominously in doubt, not just from the newer demands placed on medical education, but from its own lack of internal cohesion.

Final Years, 1900–1911

By the last quarter of the nineteenth century, medical reform had become a reality for increasing numbers of state medical boards, boards of examiners, and individual schools. The standards set in 1877 by the Illinois State Board of Health and the growing pressures for curricular reform by school administrators and concerned faculty were complemented by the establishment of scientific societies and the reorganization in 1893 of the defunct Association of American Medical Colleges. The Council on Medical Education of the American Medical Association, created in 1903, began to classify medical colleges in 1907. In 1904, only four medical colleges required baccalaureate-level work beyond high school. By 1913, eighty-four colleges required one or more years of college work; and of these, thirty-four required two or more years of collegiate work before a student could be admitted to medical school.[1] In 1901, 100 colleges held sessions from twenty-three to twenty-eight weeks; by 1914, only 2 colleges reported sessions of less than twenty-nine weeks.[2]

According to John B. Nichols, in the *Journal of the American Medical Association* in 1913, the one aspect that gave regular medicine a standing apart from sectarianism was its scientific character. "There are no sects in science, no schools of truth," he argued. "While facts of Nature are being studied out and until final certainty is attained, there may be legitimate and amicable differences of opinion in the scientific fold; but in ultimate truth there is an essential unity, and no contradictions are possible. The existence of conflicting sects and schools . . . of chemistry or astronomy or any objective science, is unthinkable; it is equally incongruous in medicine."[3] In making this assertion, Nichols admitted to many shortcomings and imperfections in regular medicine. Clearly its ranks contained individuals who in their incompetence were little more than quacks. "Low standards of medical education in the past have enabled many inadequately trained persons to obtain the legal right to practice medicine," he wrote. There were limitations to what therapeutics could accomplish, and like other mortals, physicians were neither perfect nor infallible. But only a truly scientific medicine could attain the "maximum possible truth and efficiency and the minimum of error and harmfulness." Sectarianism could not provide this. Unless it rested on a scientific foundation, utilizing the scientific method to build its knowledge base, sectarian medicine would remain narrow, tyrannical, and susceptible to error.[4]

Medicine as Applied Science

Arthur Dean Bevan, M.D., for ten years chairman of the Council on Medical Education of the American Medical Association and a staunch admirer of the German university system, recalled in an address before the Aesculapian Club of Harvard University in 1912 that the past thirty years had witnessed a revolution in medicine. "A new and great science, the science of medicine, has been born," he informed his audience, "and the change has been so rapid and so great that even those of us who are not old can reach back and touch the dark days, when medicine was not a science."[5] Scientific medicine emerged with advances in modern pathology and bacteriology, in anatomy (especially histology and embryology), and in physiology. Modern pharmacology and the laboratory sciences melded in the crucible of clinical medicine.[6]

Modern scientific medicine placed the patient at the center of study. This meant locating the medical school in a population center, surrounded by a dispensary and hospital; establishing clinical and research laboratories of anatomy, physiology, pathology, and pharmacology; and maintaining a trained staff of clinical and laboratory teachers. None of this came cheaply, and those medical schools that schemed to do it on the margin produced doctors who made little contribution to the new age. For Bevan, the German teaching clinics of Anton von Eiselsberg, Theodor Kocher, Rudolph Krause, and Friedrich von Müller stood as models for American medical departments to emulate.[7]

Bevan pointed out two immediate problems that confronted American medical education: first, the need to develop trained teachers in medicine; and second, the need to develop the appropriate affiliation between university medical departments and good hospitals. To solve the first problem, he urged adoption of the German educational model of employing full-time teachers of anatomy, physiology, and pathology who had both medical training and hospital experience. "It is a mistake to put a man direct from the laboratory sciences, no matter how brilliant, into a clinical chair," commented Bevan. "Laboratory training is most desirable but these men in addition to their laboratory training should serve their five or ten years of apprenticeship as assistants in clinical work."[8] In dealing with the second issue, he urged greater cooperation between the medical department of the university and the municipal and general hospital. Here again, examples were to be found in the affiliations that medical departments of German universities had developed with the great municipal hospitals. "It is an economic wrong for the university to conduct a hospital for the sole purpose of teaching and research, and a sociologic crime for the municipality to conduct a hospital as a boarding-house for the care of the sick without any regard for the educational and research functions of the hospital," he explained to the faculty of Harvard University. Instead, he called for a union of the two. "The hospital should provide for the care of the sick and the university should provide for the teaching and research function of the great hospital." The administrative and medical bodies each had separate functions to perform, but they could achieve their separate and mutual ends only through cooperation.[9]

Besides their affiliations with large general hospitals, university medical departments also required affiliations with more specialized hospitals such as eye and ear, infectious diseases, maternity, and orthopedic. Equally important, departments needed to appoint persons to clinical chairs who could combine teaching, hospital work, and research with private practice. "It is of course unfortunate when . . . a clinician called to a chair . . . proceeds to capitalize the reputation of the university and makes it pay handsome dividends into his own pocket," commented Bevan. "But on the other hand it would be unfortunate for American medicine if our great university clinicians were placed in a position where their services were rendered exclusively to the poor, and the well-to-do were deprived of them." Seeking the best possible solution to the problem, he again turned to the German model, believing that the clinical teacher should have the right and the opportunity to do a limited amount of private practice. To sever the clinician from practice would result in filling university chairs "with mediocre men and deprive the medical school of the services of the best brains in clinical work."[10]

Preeminent in establishing medicine as an applied science was recognizing the university as the only proper environment for mastering the fundamentals of the scientific disciplines. The spirit and method of research in the branch sciences set the standard for the successful practitioner of medicine. The rules of diagnosis and treatment were only as good as the examination of the facts and the application of the principles of anatomy, physiology, pathology, chemistry, embryology, pharmacology, and bacteriology. Only teachers engaged in research could support the needs of modern medicine. Equally important, such teachers could not be self-constituted but rather selected on the basis of their scientific attainments and advanced in rank on the merits of their teaching and research accomplishments.

In light of these new and more demanding standards, two things became obvious. First, the university was the only appropriate home for America's medical schools; and second, the real expense of medical education could not be financed through tuition and fees alone. Public tax dollars and/or private endowment furnished the only feasible schemes for meeting these costs. So long as the medical school remained the private estate of its faculty or a small number of stockholders, little public or private money would flow in to support its educational needs and objectives. As Professor Henry P. Bowditch, the organizer of Harvard's first laboratory of experimental physiology explained it, "One might as well expect the public to endow cotton mills."[11]

The opening of the Johns Hopkins Medical School in 1893 and its admissions requirement of four years of college marked a watershed in the standards for medical education and in the expectations for medical research. But the school's opening also marked something else: Its financing represented a stark contrast to existing institutions owned and operated by the faculty as private proprietary businesses. These latter institutions could no longer face the increased expenses and expectations associated with modern medical education. The German pattern of university clinics, the development of full-time teaching positions, the interaction of the medical school with other graduate departments in the university, the participation of students in ongoing research, and the emphasis on a scientific-based physician-patient relationship, became the prototype that the Johns Hopkins Medical School bequeathed in quick succession to a number of other schools.[12]

The new directions set by Johns Hopkins in admission requirements, curriculum, endowment, organization, and the role of research and clinical medicine spread across the educational landscape as schools caught the spirit of reform and sought to operate on a par with European medical standards. These included Harvard University Medical School, Yale University Medical School, Columbia University Medical School, the Department of Medicine of the University of Pennsylvania, Northwestern University Medical School, and the University of Chicago Medical School. Beneath this top echelon operated the majority of colleges whose departments of medicine could claim only nominal university affiliation (i.e., Marquette University and the Milwaukee Medical College; Loyola University and the Bennett College of Eclectic Medicine and Surgery; Union University and the Albany Medical School) and that required organizational, curricular, and fiscal restructuring. A third tier of schools, incapable of meeting new requirements, was fast disappearing from the scene through merger or outright closure. Many in this group found it difficult to form university associations and faced similar problems in introducing laboratory methods, hiring salaried teachers in the fundamental sciences, and maintaining hospitals and dispensaries to provide adequate clinical material for their students. These included most of the homeopathic and eclectic schools, as well as the remaining physio-medical colleges.[13]

The American Medical Association's Council on Medical Education attempted to realize, among its objectives, that state licensing exams should favor schools that offered training in scientific medicine. To help attain this objective, the council graded each medical school (A, B, C) on the percentage of graduates who passed state board exams; the requirement of preliminary education for applicants to medical school; the quality of the medical curriculum; the extent of plant and laboratory facilities; the quality and operation of dispensary and hospital facilities; the evidence of original research; and the quality of faculty, libraries, and teaching equipment. Although the results of the council's survey were not made public, the grading of medical colleges meant the beginning of the end for inferior schools. Colleges either merged or went out of business in the wake of these new criteria, and by the time the second nationwide inspection was published in 1910 (Flexner Report), the number of schools had already diminished by nearly 25 percent from the 1905 total. Still, of the 131 remaining medical schools in the United States in 1910, 32 were sectarian institutions: 15 homeopathic; 8 eclectic; 8 osteopathic; and 1 physio-medical.[14]

In 1905, the Association of American Medical Colleges amended its bylaws by requiring each matriculant to its sixty-eight member colleges to have a diploma from a four-year high school (or normal school) or a bachelor's degree from an approved college or university, or to pass an examination on specified branches of knowledge.[15] The association also adopted a standard curriculum of 4,000 hours for its member schools. As Samuel James of the University Medical College of Kansas City observed in his presidential address before the organization: "In my opinion, the day of unworthy medical schools is past and that it is only a matter of a few years more when they will be swallowed up by the larger institution or cease to exist entirely."[16] From then on, effective cooperation between the Association of American Medical Colleges and the American Medical Association meant the revitalization of medical education, licensing standards, and self-regulation.

Clearly, medical education was well on its way to reform before the Carnegie Foundation, under the direction of Henry S. Pritchett, selected Abraham Flexner to examine the state of medical education in the United States and Canada. Flexner, who had received his bachelor's degree from Johns Hopkins in 1886, responded with a report that resulted in commitments from a dozen or more foundations to support his recommendations. In the decades that followed, foundation monies financed a new scientific paradigm for medicine, and those regular and sectarian schools that failed to measure up moved into the backwaters where they lingered until they merged or closed. Students from nonscientific schools quickly learned there was no future for them in a marketplace controlled by state licensing boards under the influence and direction of physicians educated with an appreciation of basic research, academically based sciences, and the new directions and emphases learned from German-educated professors.[17]

With the work of the Council on Medical Education and the Association of American Medical Colleges, the efforts of state licensing boards, and the support of the Carnegie Foundation and similar funding agencies, the medical landscape changed dramatically. The number of schools declined from 160 in 1900 to 122 in 1911, and it seemed probable to observers like Arthur Dean Bevan that the United States might end up with 60 or 70 schools based on a sound university affiliation.[18]

The number of medical students in the United States showed similar declines—from 25,171 in 1900 to 19,786 in 1911 when the physios graduated their last class of students. The decrease in students attending sectarian colleges stemmed in no small measure from the enforcement of higher entrance standards, especially the requirement of one to two years of preliminary collegiate work, the replacement of the lecture mode of instruction with laboratory and clinical teaching, and the growing public intolerance toward discredited schools and cheapened standards.

The physios were by no means immune to these pressures and saw clearly the challenge these reforms meant to their very existence. Like the eclectics and homeopaths, they viewed change with suspicion, knowing all too well that allopaths were effectively controlling public opinion in matters of licensing and medical education.

Chicago Physio-Medical Institute

As noted in chapter 4, following the dissension between the trustees and faculty of the Physio-Medical Institute in Cincinnati, William H. Cook closed the doors of the school after serving twenty-five years as its dean; he moved to Chicago where he opened the Chicago Physio-Medical Institute. He took with him W. F. Tait and professors Snyder and Blair, all of whom helped to secure the school's recognition by the Illinois Board of Health. The first of its twenty-six week sessions began September 1885.

In moving the school to Chicago, Cook committed himself to strengthening physio-medicalism—not by rejecting curricular reform but by attempting to identify an appropriate niche in the medical education

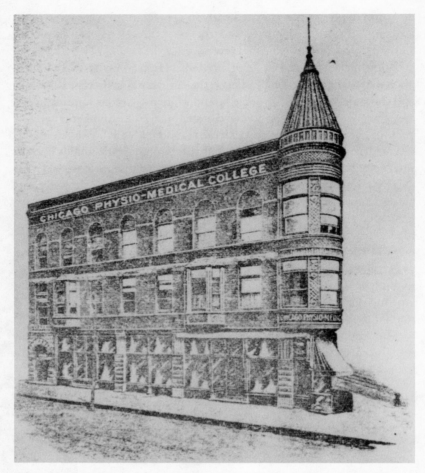

Chicago Physio-Medical College (1898). From "Chicago Physio-Medical College," *Sanative Medicine* 8 (1898): 202. Courtesy of the Lloyd Library and Museum, Cincinnati.

structure. He realized that the school could not compete with university-based medical programs, but the city with its diversity of peoples and diseases was a worthy substitute for the university's scientific laboratories. "It is becoming more and more evident," he wrote in an introductory pamphlet on the college, that "the teaching of medicine is leaving the didactic mode and taking on the form of clinics, or actual presentation on the living body." For this reason, "the larger the city, the more various and numerous will be its forms of disease, and the broader will be the medical knowledge of him who studies medicine in this city."[19]

To its many friends, the college was known as "old fountain head." George Hasty of Indiana grudgingly admitted that it deserved the title, but he accused the new school of claiming to be big enough to meet the needs of all physios. Speaking for those not attached to the Chicago institute, Hasty viewed this bravado as little more than a marketing scheme concocted by the Chicago faculty to garner greater control over reform medicine. Instead, he urged the faculty at the new institute to "do honest work and clear up [the school's] old record." There was room enough for a dozen or more physio colleges and certainly no need to assert that all the educational needs of reform medicine could be managed by a single school.[20] In truth, Hasty had never liked Cook and his faculty, believing that neither the Cincinnati institute nor its reconstituted school in Chicago "had a man in it that was regarded or recognized as a physio-medicalist." These were tough words from one who had once held a teaching position on the college's faculty.[21]

By acquiring larger hospital and clinical facilities and a training school for nurses educated in physio-medical principles, the school obtained a new charter in 1891 and changed its name to the Chicago Physio-Medical College. From 1891 to 1895 it was located at 605 West Van Buren Street, in the vicinity of Cook County Hospital, Presbyterian Hospital, Hospital for Women and Children, and the West Side Free Dispensary.[22] E. W. Lyman served as president of its board of directors, Jonas E. Roop as president of the faculty, and Hugh P. Nelson as secretary. In the school's announcement, the faculty noted their preference for retaining its old name, but "times have changed and after long deliberation . . . the faculty . . . decided to take a more modern name, and with the change of name also a change of organization." Along with the name change, the school expanded its capital stock in recognition that no medical college could pay its own way in an era of expanded curriculum and expensive laboratory facilities. Nelson urged friends of physio-medicalism to support the school through stock purchases (ten dollars per share) and scholarship certificates (fifty dollars each).[23]

The school's faculty of fourteen (by 1896 the number had increased to thirty-four), included Hugh P. Nelson in principles and practice of medicine and clinical medicine; Jonas E. Roop in obstetrics and diseases

Advertisement for the Chicago Physio-Medical College (1893). From *Physio-Medical Journal* 19 (1893): 7. Courtesy of the Lloyd Library and Museum, Cincinnati.

of women and children; Horace J. Treat in surgery, ophthalmology, and otology; William H. Cook in nervous diseases and materia medica; W. F. Tait in minor surgery and surgical anatomy; F. O. Broady in histology, pathology, and insanity; and H. A. Hadley in chemistry, toxicology, and anatomy. Each had an established private practice in Chicago. According to Roop, the faculty represented "the most conservative methods as well as the most improved and reliable means for the diagnosis and treatment of disease."[24]

The college's 1891 announcement reiterated its dedication to the physio-medical method of medication and its promise to have nothing to do with "similars" or "contraries" or with the science of probabilities. Rather, the college had raised medicine "to the rank of a true science" and an "exact knowledge" with a foundation based on the axiom that "any given property of a matter is constant." Applied to the use of medicinal substances, the action of any drug was always the same, regardless of the quantity used. Thus physio-medicalism represented a new system of medicine that taught students to be the "followers and assistants of nature" and recognized that true scientific medication consisted of purely sanative, nonpoisonous agents whose actions harmonized with nature's efforts.[25]

Instruction at the college included a combination of didactic and clinical lectures, operative recitations, quizzes, and practical demonstrations. The faculty did not undervalue didactic lectures but gave greater emphasis to work in the laboratory, dissecting room, and clinic. Lectures were given Monday through Saturday, with time allocated on Tuesday, Thursday, and Saturday for clinical and so-called "mortuary investigations."[26]

In 1895, the college moved to larger facilities at 517–19–21 Milwaukee Avenue. Later that year, the Illinois State Board of Health recognized the college in "good standing," following upgrades to its chemical laboratory and clinical department. Recognition had not been easy to obtain, and the college had been forced to engage legal counsel to argue its case. Once recognition was obtained, however, W. Francis Pechuman, M.D., secretary of the college observed: "While we have been in trouble, we have worked; it is well sometimes, to get in trouble; it sharpens the mind for better work." Physio-medicalism was "throwing off its old coat, it is putting on a new dress, but . . . with the same true heart true to a noble cause."[27]

Advertisement for the College of Medicine and Surgery, Physio-Medical, Chicago. From *Sanative Medicine* 13 (1903). Courtesy of the Lloyd Library and Museum, Cincinnati.

By 1893, more than 90 percent of American medical colleges offered a three-year program, and the top tier of schools were beginning to institute a compulsory fourth year. For the Chicago Physio-Medical College, graduation requirements in 1895 included attaining the age of twenty-one; having a good moral character; studying medicine for four years, including three full courses of lectures, the last of which was with the Chicago Physio-Medical College; passing written and oral examinations; pursuing the study of practical anatomy, including dissecting at least "two parts of the human body"; and paying in full the college fees. Tickets for the course of lectures cost sixty-five dollars; other expenses were a demonstrator's fee of ten dollars, a breakage fee of five dollars, a hospital ticket of five dollars, a matriculation fee of five dollars, and a graduation fee of thirty-five dollars.[28]

In 1897, for reasons that are not entirely clear, Cook, Tait, and Nelson withdrew from the school and organized a rival Chicago College of

Medicine and Surgery, Physio-Medical, at 322 West Eighteenth Street, with twenty-two part-time faculty.[29] Two years later, the schism ended; the two schools merged under the leadership of Nelson and became the College of Medicine and Surgery, Physio-Medical. Located now at 245–247 Ashland Boulevard, the college reported a part-time faculty of thirty-one and a college dispensary that supplied material for clinical work. The program covered four years of seven months each, with fees of $100 for the first year, $95 for the second and third years, and $110 for the fourth year. Total registration for 1900–1901 was forty-six students, with nine graduates.[30] By 1904, it claimed a faculty of forty-four, with a total registration of seventy students and eleven graduates.[31]

Physio-Medical College of Texas

In June 1883, a group of Texas physios met in Dallas to establish a state organization and adopt the platform of principles approved in 1883 by the American Association of Physio-Medical Physicians and Surgeons.[32] In 1902, the Physio-Medical College of Texas (Dallas) organized with capital stock of five thousand dollars and a faculty of twenty-six, drawn almost entirely from graduates of the Physio-Medical College of Indiana. Its first class had seven students.[33] The requirements for admission were a high school diploma (or its equivalent), or an examination in English grammar, arithmetic, elementary physics, United States history, geography, and Latin. The school offered a four-year course of twenty-six weeks each and clinical privileges at the City Hospital, St. Paul's Sanitarium, and the Buckner Home Annex or Children's Hospital. By 1905, the college had thirty-nine students, six of whom were women.[34]

At the national meeting of physio-medicals in 1907, the reformers discussed the merits of uniting the Dallas, Chicago, and Indianapolis colleges into a single institution. The effort ultimately failed because of the undercurrent of bad feelings between the Indiana and Chicago faculties. Much of this animosity stemmed from the Chicago college's earlier legal battles with the Illinois State Board of Health and the refusal of the Indianapolis school to support their colleagues in the litigation. The attitude of the Indianapolis college to the plight of its sister school, observed F. O. Broady in Dallas, "will some day be the shame of Indianapolis and a bitter memory, especially if the Chicago college goes under."[35]

The merger effort also failed due to higher enrollments at each of the colleges (the Physio-Medical College of Texas had fifty-seven students by its fifth year), and each had formed agreeable hospital connections. This was no easy task given the control the regulars maintained over tax-supported hospitals. In Indiana, for example, the college had arranged to have its students admitted to the Park Maternity Home for obstetric training. Less formal arrangements existed with the Christian Hospital, Francis Willard Hospital, and Saint Mary's Hospital. In addition, the college maintained its own small hospital of twenty beds where students obtained bedside instruction.[36] Because of similar arrangements in Dallas, the stockholders of the Physio-Medical College of Texas voted in July 1907 against merger saying that "no coalition with Indianapolis and Chicago was possible at the present time."[37] Between 1901 and 1908, the three remaining physio-medical schools graduated a combined total of 145, or approximately 19 students annually.

Not until 1908 did the Texas college finally merge with the College of Medicine and Surgery, Physio-Medical, of Chicago. No official reason was given for the decision, but it seems clear that the physios were anxious to consolidate their remaining strengths into a single college rather than dissipate them in rival schools. Clearly, the cost of medical education unsupported by public tax revenues had placed a severe strain on the supporters of reform medicine. The merger did not include the Indiana college since it had announced its closing in 1909. Increased costs and the college's inability to obtain access to the city's hospital wards had all but doomed its future.

Still, matters did not improve for the sole remaining physio school. In April 1909, Abraham Flexner visited the Chicago college as part of his examination of medical education in the United States and Canada. He found that the published entrance requirements satisfied the interpretation of the law, but a search of office records failed to produce any credentials for the students presently enrolled. The teaching staff consisted of forty-two individuals, thirty-three of whom were professors, serving thirty-three students. Flexner considered the equipment "very meager" and the college's clinical facilities equally so; only 167 patients (half of whom were surgical) had registered in its hospital that year, and only 250 outpatients had used its dispensary. For its total educational program, the school relied on fees that Flexner estimated at only $2,935.[38]

The physio-medical college was one of fourteen medical schools operating in Chicago at the time of Flexner's visit, prompting him to call the city "the plague spot of the country." All but one of the fourteen schools held the status of "good standing" by the Illinois state board, but Flexner felt that only Rush, Northwestern, and the College of Physicians and Surgeons deserved the status; and of those, only Rush (which affiliated with the University of Chicago in 1898) was secure in its entrance requirements, teaching, and laboratory facilities. The entire situation, he concluded, presented the city's medical community with "a rare opportunity for educational statesmanship."[39]

In 1911, fourteen graduates of the College of Medicine and Surgery, Physio-Medical took the state boards; only four passed. This represented a 71.4 percent failure rate, the third worst in the country, followed by the University of West Tennessee Medical Department and the Hospital Medical College in Atlanta.[40] In 1911, the last remaining college of reformed medicine was absorbed by the Chicago College of Medicine and Surgery (eclectic).[41] With its absorption, the seventy-two year history of physio-medicalism ended quietly. Its leaders, once vocal and outspoken in their advocacy of botanic medicine, fell mute under the critical eyes of the Association of American Medical Colleges, the American Medical Association, state licensing boards, and the increasingly strident demands of academic medicine. In 1917, the Chicago College of Medicine and Surgery was purchased by the Loyola University School of Medicine.

A Backward Glance

For all their pretense to reform, the physios did not fare as well as either the homeopaths or the eclectics in the competition for patients and students; nor did any of the sectarian groups compete successfully with allopathy once regular medicine chose to reform. In fact, the physios had little with which to console themselves. Compared with eclectics and homeopaths, they produced fewer physicians and far fewer textbooks and medical journals. Moreover, many physios chose to practice under banners other than their own, and fewer still sent students to their physio-medical colleges.[42] Because of their smaller numbers, they were forced to rely on eclectic and regular pharmaceutical companies as the principal sources of their medicines. This they did grudgingly, accusing the eclectics of backsliding in the use of harsh medicines, particularly in the years following the work of Koch and Pasteur in germ theory.[43]

On the positive side, the physios were successful in publishing advice books and pamphlets on health and hygiene. Together with the eclectics, they produced a genre of literature that projected a very traditional and religious approach that carried considerable authority in Victorian America. Authors drew from a wealth of folk and domestic medical literature; from the quasi-scientific theories of phrenology and mesmerism; from grahamism and perfectionist tendencies that had earlier influenced adherents of the abolition, prohibition, and peace movements; from the cleansing and kindly regimens of hydropathy and Thomsonism; and from religious themes that were strikingly protestant in tone and in outcome. Here could be found the canon of medical sectarianism—a uniquely American literature in its ritual, its rejection of imported theories, its appeal to volunteerism, its deliberate protestantism, and its millennial expectancy.[44]

The physios were outwardly proud of their past and always anxious to recount the efforts of earlier stalwarts to fight "old school" medicine. They were also not averse to self-criticism. "We have not enough 'loaves and fishes' and don't know how to work miracles," admitted Ohio physio John W. Shockey in the *Physio-Medical Record* of 1906. "We have too many doctors who have no conviction and no courage if they did have them, hence, they don't amount to a damn."[45] Others blamed their troubles on those among their ranks who had deviated from accepted practice, using such alternative treatments as static electricity instead of relying on a good emetic.[46] True physios held firm to the belief that the sheet anchor of their system was the emetic. "I was in a medical conversation," wrote E. M. Haggard, M.D., in 1906, "and there was an individual . . . who said that in the last year he had given 1500 emetics and that . . . represented [all] what was known as Physio-Medicalism."[47]

Generalizations are hard to make when looking at the curricula of medical schools in the late nineteenth and early twentieth centuries. Because of the number and variety of schools, and because of the wide disparity in the caliber of instruction, available texts, equipment, and facilities, content of instruction is simply too difficult to measure. Among both regular and sectarian schools wide variations existed in time medical students spent to obtain degrees. Certainly there was a lack of uniformity in the curricula. According to George H. Simmons, M.D., speaking before the Medical Department of Drake University in 1904, medical schools offered anywhere from 200 to 1,248 hours in anatomy, 96 to 450 hours in physiology, 176 to 652 hours in chemistry, 45 to 364 hours in bacteriology, and 54 to 512 hours in pathology. Similarly, the time spent in the clinical areas varied from 64 to 1,168 hours in surgery, 140 to 1,232 in medicine, and 67 to 320 hours in obstetrics. Even worse, many colleges simply ignored clinical, hospital, and dispensary work, and sometimes even excluded instruction in physiology, bacteriology, pathology, and histology.[48]

Some medical historians have argued that sectarian medical education differed in no great degree from regular schools.[49] This was certainly true among the medical colleges not affiliated with universities, and it proved to be no less true among the physios even though they tried hard to stress their own particular brand of medicine.[50] For example, for its 1891–92 session, the Chicago Physio-Medical College listed a combination of sectarian and regular texts for its incoming class. Interestingly, only six of the seventy required or recommended texts could be classified botanic or reform literature.

One could argue, therefore, that those mainstream texts in the curriculum served as a source of authority and, as such, acted as a conservative force on the school's more idiosyncratic practices. The problem for the physios, however, was not their choice of texts but their inability to support textbook instruction with adequate laboratory and clinical experience. In both areas, they fell short due to their fragile financial structure and the control that regulars held over most public hospitals and clinics.

As more and more regular schools succeeded in re-engineering their organizational and funding structures, sectarians found themselves continually frustrated by their failure to keep pace. Lacking funds to support full-time faculty, laboratory assistants, and equipment, and unable to negotiate much needed hospital arrangements for their students, they faced the ominous reality of reorganization, merger, or extinction. True, they often spoke the language of the new scientific medicine, but few had the financial ability, the opportunity, or the willpower, to carry their aspirations into reality. Worse yet, enrollments, endowments, and state tax dollars moved perceptibly toward the more stable university-based programs.

Despite pretenses, the physios never felt at ease with the expectations of the new age. Having prided themselves in their native roots and herbs and in a commitment to a domestic practice based on a regimen of kindly medicines, they were in no position—intellectual or financial—to manage the changes that scientific medicine demanded. All but a few physios viewed laboratory science and experimental medicine as foreign and elitist, and only grudgingly did they incorporate these components into their curricula. Their inability to build a strong financial base and their continued admission of students who lacked preliminary education, including work in the basic sciences, precluded any hope that the quality of their students—or the quality of their instruction—would improve. The physios struggled unsuccessfully to provide the additional staff required for laboratory-based education; no doubt they would have preferred to be left alone, to exist on their own terms, and to change at their own speed. But the choices were not theirs to make.

There were other reasons behind the failure of the physios. By fault or by design, nineteenth-century botanic reformers were ideologues first and physicians second, and they seemed to move through a succession of moods as they sought to reconcile their democratic beliefs with the art of the possible. The grandeur of their aims became an obsessive preoccupation that all too often fragmented personal and professional friendships. As Calvin Newton knew only too well, "Differences of opinion, coupled with almost unconquerable obstinacy in maintaining them on small points" defined both their private and public sentiments. This character flaw tended over time to destroy their claims, dull the attractiveness of their ideas, and blur their vision.[51] One of the best descriptions of these nineteenth-century medical reformers came from the eclectic John M. Scudder who wrote: "They were very war-like, pugnacious as snapping turtles, but they had abundant cause for it; they were Ishmaelites, and every man's hand was against them, and they were inclined to turn their hands against other people."[52] Almost any of the various bands of botanic reformers, including the physios, fit this description.

Too often, however, we are tempted to view medicine from the perspective of our present age and fail to understand that the public's expectations for the late nineteenth- and early twentieth-century physician were not the same as they are today. In the period that encompasses the history of physio-medicalism, the ability to diagnose human ills far exceeded the ability to successfully treat them. Even with their limitations, the physios left behind a respectable legacy. Though despised by regulars, their graduates received a modicum of training and, upon graduation, served honorably as primary care providers. Unlike the eclectics and homeopaths, none achieved an international, much less a national reputation since scientific preeminence was never a part of their professional identity. Instead, they served as respected and respectable practitioners to an appreciative patient population. In rural and small-town America, and among urban working classes fresh from the American heartland, they provided a level of health care that, while distinctively simplistic, nativistic in its suspicions of foreign ideas and influences, and protestant in its democratic biases, continued an herbal tradition that held true to its Thomsonian origins and to family practice.

Through much of the nineteenth century, the public had no great affinity to regular medicine, preferring instead to judge healers more by their reputations than by their schooling or by their systems of therapeutics. Domestic and traditional folk medicine, Shaker medicine, Thomsonism, homeopathy, eclecticism, physio-medicalism, and various forms of nondescript healing practices competed in the medical marketplace of rural and small-town America. Herb cures carried no less credibility in American households because of their Indian, Shaker, or Thomsonian origins. The remedies prepared by these alternative healers worked about as well as their patients expected. In the end, the physios managed a medical education system that fostered the creation of general practitioners and evinced from patients a confidence in their sectarian differences. They were firm in their public attachment to older theories, unapologetic in their disagreements with allopathy, and millenarian in their view of the ultimate judgment of history.

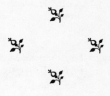

Notes

Introduction

1. "An Address to the Public," *Physio-Medical Journal* 9 (1883): 184.

1. The Medical Language

1. Martin Kaufman, "American Medical Education," in *The Education of American Physicians*, ed. Ronald Numbers (Berkeley: University of California Press, 1980), 10–11; Joseph F. Kett, *The Formation of the American Medical Profession: The Role of Institutions, 1750–1860* (New Haven: Yale University Press, 1968), chapter 3; Kenneth M. Ludmerer, *Learning to Heal: The Development of American Medical Education* (New York: Basic, 1985), chapter 1; Saul Jarcho, "The Legacy of British Medicine to American Medicine, 1800–1850," *Proceedings of the Royal Society of Medicine* 68 (1975): 25; Martin Kaufman, *American Medical Education: The Formative Years, 1765–1910* (Westport, Conn.: Greenwood, 1976), 36–56.

2. John Harley Warner, *The Therapeutic Perspective: Medical Practice, Knowledge, and Identity in America, 1820–1885* (Cambridge: Harvard University Press, 1986), 13.

3. E. H. Ackerknecht, *Medicine at the Paris Hospital, 1794–1848* (Baltimore: Johns Hopkins University Press, 1967), 5–12, 101; George Rosen, "The Philosophy of Ideology and the Emergence of Modern Medicine in France," *Bulletin of the History of Medicine* 20 (1946): 328–39.

4. William G. Rothstein, "The Botanical Movements and Orthodox Medicine," in *Other Healers: Unorthodox Medicine in America,* ed. Norman Gevitz (Baltimore: Johns Hopkins University Press, 1988), 38–39.

5. [Committee on Education], "Report," *Transactions of the American Medical Association* 1 (1848): 236–38.

6. Ibid., 243–44.

7. Ibid., 246–47.

8. Morris Fishbein, "History of the American Medical Association," *Journal of the American Medical Association* 132 (1946): 637, 699–700.

9. Ludmerer, *Learning to Heal,* 20, 61, 239.

10. W. T. Ridenour, "The Relation of Regular Medicine to the Pathies of the Day," *Transactions of the Ohio State Medical Society* 30 (1875): 50.

11. Abraham Flexner, *Medical Education in the United States and Canada; A Report to the Carnegie Foundation on the Advancement of Teaching* (New York: Carnegie Foundation, 1910), 156.

12. John S. Haller, Jr., "The Decline of Bloodletting: A Study in Nineteenth Century Ratiocinations," *Southern Medical Journal* 79 (1986): 469–75.

13. I. M. Comings, "Prospective Reform in Irregular Medical Sects," *Physio-Medical Journal* 7 (1881): 175; "The Great Pill Maker," *Physio-Medical Journal* 7 (1881): 61.

14. William H. Cook, *The Physio-Medical Dispensatory. A Treatise on the Principles and Practice of Physio-Medical Surgery; For the Use of Students and Practitioners* (Cincinnati: Moore, Wilstach, Keys, 1857), 7.

15. Quoted in Joseph M. Thurston, "Medical Philosophers and Medical Science," *Physio-Medical Journal* 14 (1888): 333; Samuel C. F. Hahnemann, *Oreganon of Homoeopathic Medicine* (New York: Radde, 1843), 68. See also chapter four ("Transcendental Medicine"), in John S. Haller, Jr., *American Medicine in Transition, 1840–1910* (Urbana: University of Illinois Press, 1981), 100–149.

16. R. Gibson Miller, "A Synopsis of Homoeopathic Philosophy," *Journal of Homoeopathics* 4 (1900): 194–214; Harris L. Coulter, *Divided Legacy: A History of Schism in Medical Thought,* vol. 3, *Science and Ethics in Medicine: 1800–1914* (Washington, D.C.: Wehawken Book Co., 1973), 5–58, 328–56; J. C. Reeve, "Some of the Latest Systems of Medicine," *Transactions of the Ohio State Medical Society* (1885): 45–46.

17. Harris L. Coulter, "Homeopathic Influences in Nineteenth Century Allopathic Therapeutics: A Historical and Philosophical Study," *Journal of the American Institute of Homeopathy* 65 (1972): 139–48.

18. Thurston, "Medical Philosophers and Medical Science," 337; Gottlieb Heinrich Jahr, *Hull's Jahr; A New Manual of Homeopathic Practice* (New York: W. Radde, 1862), 542–48.

19. J. M. Toner, "Statistical Sketch of the Medical Profession in the United States," *Indiana Journal of Medicine* 4 (1873): 4–5.

20. Judith M. Taylor, "Early Botanists and the Introduction of Drug Specifics," *Bulletin of the New York Academy of Medicine* 60 (1979): 685; Wyndham B. Blanton, *Medicine in Virginia in the Seventeenth Century* (Richmond: William Byrd, 1930), 100–101, 105–13; Wade Boyle, *Herb Doctors: Pioneers in Nineteenth-Century American Botanical Medicine and a History of the Eclectic Medical Institute of Cincinnati* (East Palestine, Ohio: Buckeye Naturopathic Press, 1988), ii; John S. Haller, Jr., *Medical Protestants: The Eclec-*

tics in American Medicine, 1825–1939 (Carbondale: Southern Illinois University Press, 1994), 8–9.

21. Catherine Wisswaesser, "Roots and Ramifications of Medicinal Herbs in 18th Century North America," *Transactions and Studies, College of Physicians of Philadelphia* 44 (1977): 196; George E. Gifford, Jr., "Medicine and Natural History—Crosscurrents in Philadelphia in the Nineteenth Century," *Transactions and Studies, College of Physicians of Philadelphia* 45 (1978): 139–40; Lyman H. Butterfield, ed., *Letters of Benjamin Rush*, 2 vols. (Princeton, N.J.: Princeton University Press, 1951), 2:185; Ann Leighton, *Early American Gardens: For Meate or Medicine* (Worcester: American Antiquarian Society, 1970).

22. John Uri Lloyd, "Concerning the American Materia Medica," *Eclectic Medical Journal* 94 (1934): 3.

23. David L. Cowan, "The Boston Editions of Nicholas Culpeper," *Journal of the History of Medicine* 11 (1956): 156–65; Gordon H. Jones, "Medical and Scientific Books in Colonial Virginia," *Bulletin of the History of Medicine* 40 (1966): 156–57; Patricia Ann Watson, *The Angelical Conjunction: The Preacher-Physicians of Colonial New England* (Knoxville: University of Tennessee Press, 1991); Philip Cash, Eric H. Christianson, and J. Worth Estes, eds., *Medicine in Colonial Massachusetts, 1620–1820* (Boston: Colonial Society of Massachusetts, 1980); J. Worth Estes and David M. Goodman, *The Changing Humors of Portsmouth: The Medical Biography of an American Town, 1623–1983* (Boston: Francis A. Countway Library of Medicine, 1986); Robert I. Goler and Pascal James Imperato, eds., *Early American Medicine: A Symposium* (New York: Fraunces Tavern Museum, 1987); John Scarborough, ed., *Folklore and Folk Medicines* (Madison: American Institute of the History of Medicine, 1987).

24. C. N. Harold, "Alumni Address," *Physio-Medical Journal* 12 (1886): 215; Rothstein, "Botanical Movements and Orthodox Medicine," 42–45; J. Worth Estes, "Samuel Thomson Rewrites Hippocrates," in *Medicine and Healing: The Dublin Seminar for New England Folklife Annual Proceedings 1990*, ed. Peter Benes (Boston: Boston University Press, 1992), 113–29.

25. Samuel Thomson, *New Guide to Health; Or, Botanic Family Physician, Containing a Complete System of Practice Upon a Plan Entirely New: With a Description of the Vegetables Made Use of, and Directions for Preparing and Administering Them to Cure Disease* (Boston: J. Howe, 1831), 4.

26. Morris Mattson, *The American Vegetable Practice; Or, a New and Improved Guide to Health Designed for the Use of Families*, 2 vols. (Boston: Daniel L. Hale, 1841), 1:162.

27. Thomson, *New Guide to Health*, 9–10, 13; L. F. Kebler, "United States Patents Granted for Medicines During the Pioneer Years of the Patent Office," *Journal of the American Pharmaceutical Association* 24 (1935): 485–89; James M. Ball, "Samuel Thomson (1769–1843) and His Patented 'System' of Medicine," *Annals of Medical History* 7 (1925): 144–48.

28. Thomson, *New Guide to Health*, 43.

29. Ibid., 10–11, 18. See also John S. Haller, Jr., "The History of Tartar Emetic in the 19th Century Materia Medica," *Bulletin of the History of Medicine* 44 (1975): 235–57; John S. Haller, Jr., "Samson of the Materia Medica: Medical Theory and the Use and Abuse of Calomel in 19th Century America," *Pharmacy in History* 12 (1971): 27–34, 67–76.

30. Warner, *The Therapeutic Perspective*, 12.

31. Thomson, *New Guide to Health*, 25.

32. Ibid., 40–66; Philip D. Jordan, "The Secret Six: An Inquiry Into the Basic Materia Medica of the Thomsonian System of Botanic Medicine," *Ohio State Archaeological and Historical Quarterly* 52 (1943): 350; Frank G. Halstead, "A First-Hand Account of a Treatment by Thomsonian Medicine in the 1830s," *Bulletin of the History of Medicine* 10 (1941): 681–85.

33. John Shockey, "The History of Physio-Medicalism," *Physio-Medical Record* 9 (1906): 173; William Coolidge Lane, "Dr. Benjamin Waterhouse and Harvard University," *Publications*, Cambridge Historical Society, 4 (1909): 5–22; Josiah Charles Trent, "Benjamin Waterhouse (1754–1846)," *Journal of the History of Medicine* 1 (1946): 357–64. See also Stephen Nissenbaum, *Sex, Diet, and Debility in Jacksonian America: Sylvester Graham and Health Reform* (Westport, Conn.: Greenwood, 1980).

34. Alex Berman, "The Impact of the Nineteenth Century Botanico-Medical Movement on American Pharmacy and Medicine" (Ph.D. diss., University of Wisconsin, 1954), 31; Estes, "Samuel Thomson Rewrites Hippocrates," 125–26; Joanna Smith Weinstock, "Samuel Thomson's Botanic System: Alternative Medicine in Early-Nineteenth Century Vermont," *Vermont History* 56 (1988): 5–22.

35. E. Anthony, "Physio-Medicalism and Progress," *Physio-Medical Journal* 12 (1886): 227; Ball, "Samuel Thomson (1769–1843) and His Patented 'System' of Medicine," 144–49; Frederick C. Waite, "Thomsonianism in Ohio," *Ohio State Archaeological and Historical Quarterly* 44 (1940): 323; William L. Johnson, "To the Editor," *Thomsonian Recorder* 50 (1837): 228; Alva Curtis, *A Fair Examination and Criticism of All the Medical Systems in Vogue* (Cincinnati: Printed for the Proprietor, 1865), 193.

36. Alex Berman, "The Thomsonian Movement and Its Relation to American Pharmacy and Medicine," *Bulletin of the History of Medicine* 25 (1951): 417, 420; Philip D. Jordan, "Botanic Medicine in the Western Country," *Ohio State Medical Journal* 40 (1944): 143–46, 240–42.

37. Ackerknecht, *Medicine at the Paris Hospital*, 101, 104–13.

38. Thurston, "Medical Philosophers and Medical Science," 341; Robley Dunglison, *History of Medicine, From the Earliest Ages to the Commencement of the Nineteenth Century* (Philadelphia: Lindsay and Blakistan, 1872), 166.

39. Curtis, *A Fair Examination and Criticism of All the Medical Systems*, 105.

40. Lloyd, "Concerning the American Materia Medica," 10–11.

41. William G. Rothstein, *American Physicians in the Nineteenth Century: From Sects to Science* (Baltimore: Johns Hopkins University Press, 1972), 223–24.

42. J. H. Beal, "Some Aspects of Eclecticism as They Appear to a Majority of Pharmacists," *Eclectic Medical Journal* 91 (1931): 434–35.

43. Herbert T. Webster, "Not the Name, But the Game," *California Eclectic Medical Journal* 34 (1913): 36.

44. Lloyd, "Concerning the American Materia Medica," 12–14.

45. Ibid., 12.

46. "National Confederation of Eclectic Medical Colleges, 1905," LLM, coll. 3, vol. 24, Scrapbook. n.p.

47. Henry I. Bowditch, "The Past, Present, and Future Treatment of Homeopathy, Eclecticism and Kindred Delusions," *Transactions of the Rhode Island Medical Society*, 3 (1885), 300.

48. Edward Jackson, "Against Sectarianism in Medicine," *Proceedings of the Philadelphia County Medical Society* 10 (1889): 274–75, 277.

49. George Hasty, "Regular or Right, Which?" *Physio-Medical Journal* 15 (1889): 7–9.

2. Thomson's Progeny

1. Alex Berman, "The Thomsonian Movement and Its Relation to American Pharmacy and Medicine," *Bulletin of the History of Medicine* 25 (1951): 424.

2. E. Anthony, "Physio-Medicalism and Progress," *Physio-Medical Journal* 12 (1886): 227.

3. Anthony, "Physio-Medicalism and Progress," 232–33.

4. Worthington Hooker, *Dissertation on the Respect Due to the Medical Profession, and the Reasons Why It is Not Awarded by the Community* (Norwich: J. G. Cooley, 1844), 15; Worthington Hooker, *Physician and Patient; Or, A Practical View of the Mutual Duties, Relations, and Interests of the Medical Profession and the Community* (New York: Baker and Scribner, 1849), 119; Alex Berman, "Neo-Thomsonianism in the United States," *Journal of the History of Medicine* 2 (1956): 133.

5. J. Jackson, "Quackery," *New England Botanic Medical and Surgical Journal* 2 (1848): 35.

6. Horton Howard, *An Improved System of Botanic Medicine Founded Upon Correct Principles; Comprising a Complete Treatise on the Materia Medica* (Cincinnati: Kost, Bigger and Hart, 1832), 15; Alex Berman, "A Striving for Scientific Respectability: Some American Botanics and the Nineteenth Century Plant Materia Medica," *Bulletin of the History of Medicine* 30 (1956): 8.

7. Harvey D. Little, "Editor's Address to the Reader," *The Eclectic, and Medical Botanist* 1 (1833): 11–12.

8. Harvey D. Little, "Dr. H. Howard," *The Eclectic, and Medical Botanist* 1 (1833): 145.

9. Horton Howard, "To the Public," *The Eclectic, and Medical Botanist* 1 (1833): 209.

10. Benjamin Rush, *Medical Inquiries and Observations*, 2d ed., 4 vols. (Philadelphia: J. Conrad and Co., 1789), 1:276; Richard H. Shryock, "The Medical Reputation of Benjamin Rush: Contrasts Over Two Centuries," *Bulletin of the History of Medicine* 45 (1971): 507–52.

11. Howard, *An Improved System of Botanic Medicine Founded Upon Correct Physiological Principles*, 3–4.

12. Ibid., 6.

13. Ibid., 5–6.

14. The Southern Illinois University School of Medicine Library owns a copy handsigned by the executors and dated October 1839. See signed statement by "Executors of Horton Howard," in Horton Howard, *An Improved System of Botanic Medicine: Founded Upon Correct Physiology; Together With an Illustration of the New Theory of Medicine*, 3rd ed., 3 vols. (Columbus, Ohio: Published by the Proprietors, 1836).

15. Elisha Smith, *The Botanic Physician; Being a Compendium of the Practice of Physic, Upon Botanical Principles* (New York: Murphy and Bingham, 1830); Berman, "A Striving for Scientific Respectability: Some American Botanics and the Nineteenth Century Plant Materia Medica," 9–11; Alexander Wilder, *A History of Medicine: A Brief Outline of*

Medical History From the Earliest Historic Period With an Extended Account of the Various Sects of Physicians and New Schools of Medicine in Later Centuries (Augusta, Maine: Maine Farmer Publishing, 1904), 445. See also William Buchan, *Domestic Medicine, Or, A Treatise on the Prevention and Cure of Diseases by Regimen and Simple Medicine* (Edinburgh: Balfour, Auld and Smellie, 1797); Robert Thomas, *A Treatise on Domestic Medicine* (New York: Collins, 1822); James Thacher, *The American New Dispensatory* (Boston: Thomas B. Wait, 1813); Constantine S. Rafinesque, *Medical Flora: Or, Manual of the Medical Botany of the United States of North America,* 2 vols. (Philadelphia: Atkinson and Alexander, 1828–30); and Samuel Henry, *A New and Complete Family Herbal* (New York: Samuel Henry, 1814).

16. See Morris Mattson, *The American Vegetable Practice, Or, A New and Improved Guide to Health, Designed for the Use of Families,* 2 vols. (Boston: Daniel L. Hale, 1841).

17. Berman, "A Striving for Scientific Respectability," 16; Samuel Thomson, *The Thomsonian Materia Medica or Botanic Family Physician; Comprising a Philosophical Theory, the Natural Organization and Assumed Principles of Animal and Vegetable Life: To Which are Added the Description of Plants* (Albany: J. Munsell, 1841).

18. Berman, "Neo-Thomsonianism in the United States," 134.

19. Samuel Thomson, "Please to Take Notice," *Thomsonian Recorder* 4 (1836): 187. See also Alex Berman, "The Thomsonian Movement and Its Relation to American Pharmacy and Medicine," 426; Jonathan Forman, "Dr. Alva Curtis in Columbus, The Thomsonian Recorder and Columbus' First Medical School," *Ohio State Archaeological and Historical Quarterly* 51 (1942): 337.

20. Charles A. Stafford, "The Hero as a Doctor—Dr. Samuel Thomson," *Physio-Medical Journal* 16 (1890): 130–32, 135.

21. "Thomsonian Books," *Thomsonian Recorder* 2 (1834): 208; James O. Breeden, "Thomsonianism in Virginia," *Virginia Magazine of History and Biography* 82 (1974): 154–55; Joseph F. Kett, *The Formation of the American Medical Profession: The Role of Institutions, 1730–1860* (New Haven: Yale University Press, 1968), 125–26.

22. Breeden, "Thomsonianism in Virginia," 173.

23. Alva Curtis, "Form of a Thomsonian License," *Thomsonian Recorder* 5 (1837): 239.

24. Waite, "Thomsonianism in Ohio," 325; Breeden, "Thomsonianism in Virginia," 173.

25. Alva Curtis, "Remarks," *Thomsonian Recorder* 5 (1837): 229.

26. Alva Curtis, "Botanico-Medical School," *Thomsonian Recorder* 5 (1836): 30.

27. Curtis, "Botanico-Medical School," 30; Benjamin Smith Barton, *Elements of Botany; Or, Outlines of the Natural History of Vegetables* (Philadelphia: Printed for the Author, 1803); Amos Eaton, *Manual of Botany, for North America: Containing Generic and Specific Descriptions of the Indigenous Plants and Common Cultivated Exotics, Growing North of the Gulf of Mexico,* 5th ed. (Albany: Websters and Skinners, 1829).

28. E. H. Stockwell, Introductory Lecture to the Medical Class of the Physiopathic College," *Physio-Medical Recorder and Surgical Journal* 19 (1851): 322; W. H. Cook, "Higher Education," *Sanative Medicine* 4 (1894): 494; Frederick C. Waite, "American Sectarian Medical Colleges Before the Civil War," *Bulletin of the History of Medicine* 19 (1946): 152.

29. Stockwell, "Introductory Lecture to the Medical Class of the Physiopathic College," 322; Otto Juettner, *Daniel Drake and His Followers: Historical and Biographical Sketches* (Cincinnati: Harvey, 1909), 109–10; Breeden, "Thomsonianism in Virginia," 172. The Botanico-Medical College in Cincinnati was the second chartered sectarian

medical school in the United States, following the Medical Department of Worthington College (eclectic), also in Ohio, and chartered in 1830.

30. Jerry Bryan Lincecum and Edward Hake Phillips, eds., *Adventures of a Frontier Naturalist: The Life and Times of Dr. Gideon Lincecum* (College Station, Tex.: Texas A&M University Press, 1994), chapters 5 and 10. See also "Communications," *Botanico-Medical Recorder* 8 (1839–40): 116–18, 304–6; 9 (1840–41): 81–85, 130; 10 (1841–42): 130; 12 (1843–44): 83–84; 13 (1844–45): 4–5.

31. Curtis, "Botanico Medical School," 395–96.

32. "Doctor Alva Curtis," *Physio-Medical Journal* 7 (1881): 33–36.

33. "Professors of the Physio-Medical College, Cincinnati, Ohio," *Physio-Medical Recorder and Surgical Journal* 17 (1849): 197.

34. "Doctor Alva Curtis," 36–37.

35. J. Osgood, "The Opposition Movement—Additional Views," *New England Botanic Medical and Surgical Journal* 2 (1848): 91.

36. Galei [pseud.], "History of Medical Reform in New England," *New England Botanic Medical and Surgical Journal* 5 (1851): 17.

37. J. Brown, "In the Field," *Physiologico-Medical Recorder and Surgical Journal* 18 (1850): 165–66; E. H. Stockwell, "Agents of the P.-M. College," *Physio-Medical Recorder and Surgical Journal* 18 (1850): 167. (These two journals are the same, only identified by different titles in these two issues.)

38. Anthony, "Physio-Medicalism and Progress," 228.

39. Announcement, *New England Botanic Medical and Surgical Journal* 5 (1851): 346; Stockwell, "Introductory Lecture on the Medical Class of the Physopathic College," 322.

40. Cook, "Higher Education," 4:495; "Doctor Alva Curtis," 37–38; W. H. Cook, "The Old P.-M. College," *Physio-Medical Recorder* 34 (1870): 85–87.

41. Cook, "Higher Education," 495.

42. Ibid., 516.

43. Ibid., William H. Cook, *The Physio-Medical Dispensatory: A Treatise on Therapeutics, Materia Medica, and Pharmacy, in Accordance With the Principles of Physiological Medication* (Cincinnati: W. H. Cook, 1869).

44. Cook, "Higher Education," 517.

45. Ibid., 519.

46. Ibid.

47. Ibid., 495.

48. William H. Cook, "Diplomas Honorable and Dishonorable," *Cincinnati Medical Gazette: A Journal of Medical Reform* 1 (1877): 165.

49. William H. Cook, "Resignation of Professor Curtis," *Physio-Medical Recorder* 26 (1862): 114.

50. Editor, "Editorial Miscellany," *Physio-Medical Recorder* 23 (1858): 88.

51. Letter quoted in Cook, "Resignation of Professor Curtis," 114.

52. Editor, "Editorial Miscellany," *Physio-Medical Recorder* 23 (1858): 200.

53. "Dr. Curtis's Tour of the States," *Physio-Medical Recorder* 12 (1858): 212.

54. Cook, "Resignation of Professor Curtis," 114.

55. W. H. Cook, "Shall It Be Honor or Dishonor?" *Cincinnati Medical Gazette: A Journal of Medical Reform* 55 (1881): 131.

56. "Doctor Alva Curtis," 37–38; Cook, "Higher Education," 495; Levi Hawkins, "Address on Alva Curtis," *Sanative Medicine* 2 (1893): 258.

57. Alva Curtis, *The Provocation and the Reply; Or, Allopathy Versus Physio-Medicalism in a Review of Prof. M. B. Wright's Remarks at the Dedication of the Cincinnati New Hospital, January 8th, 1869* (Cincinnati: Published for the Proprietor, 1870), 147.

58. Ibid., 154; Alva Curtis, *Allopathy and Physio-Medication Contrasted* (Cincinnati: By the Author, 1867), 7.

59. Anthony, "Physio-Medicalism and Progress," 229.

3. Years of Challenge

1. William H. Cook, "Higher Education," *Sanative Medicine* 4 (1894): 493–94; William H. Cook, "Physio-Medicalism Assailed and Defended," *Sanative Medicine* 5 (1895): 4.

2. Alex Berman, "Neo-Thomsonianism in the United States," *Journal of the History of Medicine* 2 (1956): 139–40.

3. Circular, "Southern Botanico-Medical College," *New England Botanic Medical and Surgical Journal* 2 (1848): 245; Circular, "Southern Botanico-Medical College," *Southern Medical Reformer* 1 (1845): 245.

4. "Reform Medical Practice," *Physio-Medical Recorder* 23 (1858): 172; Faculty of the Reform Medical College of Georgia, *The Reform-Medical Practice: With a History of Medicine, From the Earliest Period to the Present Time, and a Synopsis of Principles on Which the New Practice is Founded* (Macon, Ga.: M. S. Thomson, 1857).

5. "Isaac Miller Comings, M.D.," *Physio-Medical Journal* 17 (1891): 288–91; William H. Cook, "Professor I. M. Comings, A.M., M.D.," *Physio-Medical Recorder* 36 (1872): 9–13.

6. I. M. Comings, "Address," *Southern Medical Reformer* 1 (1845): 187.

7. "Isaac Miller Comings, M.D.," 288–91; Cook, "Professor I. M. Comings, A.M., M.D.," 9–13.

8. Masthead, *Southern Medical Reformer* 1 (1845): cover.

9. H. M. Price, "Defining our Position," *Southern Medical Reformer* 1 (1845): 27–28.

10. D. L. Terry, "Letter," *Southern Medical Reformer* 1 (1845): 25; H. M. Price, "Dr. A. Curtis," *Southern Medical Reformer* 1 (1845): 29.

11. "Thomsonism North," *Physio-Medical Recorder* 22 (1858): 131.

12. Berman, "Neo-Thomsonianism in the United States," 140; Frederick C. Waite, "American Sectarian Medical Colleges Before the Civil War," *Bulletin of the History of Medicine* 19 (1946): 153; E. Anthony, "Physio-Medicalism and Progress," *Physio-Medical Journal* 12 (1886): 229; Frederick C. Waite, "The First Sectarian Medical School in New England, at Worcester (1848–1859), and Its Relation to Thomsonianism," *New England Journal of Medicine* 207 (1932): 985; James M. Ball, "Samuel Thomson (1769–1843) and His Patented 'System' of Medicine," *Annals of Medical History* 7 (1925): 149–50.

13. "Alabama Medical Institute at Wetumpka," *Southern Medical Reformer* 1 (1845): 187.

14. James Massey, "Communication," *Southern Medical Reformer* 1 (1845): 250–51.

15. Circular, "Botanico-Medical College of Memphis, Tennessee," *Worcester Journal of Medicine* 7 (1852): 192–93.

16. Berman, "Neo-Thomsonianism in the United States," 149; Waite, "American Sectarian Medical Colleges Before the Civil War," 156.

17. "Southern Department," *New England Botanic Medical and Surgical Journal* 1 (1847): 131–32; John S. Haller, Jr., *Medical Protestants: The Eclectics in American Medicine, 1825–1939* (Carbondale: Southern Illinois University Press, 1993), 66–93.

18. "Scientific and Eclectic Medical Institute of Virginia," *New England Botanic Medical and Surgical Journal* 1 (1847): 272.

19. Circular, "Scientific and Eclectic Medical Institute of Virginia," *New England Botanic Medical and Surgical Journal* 2 (1848): 287.

20. Circular, "Scientific and Eclectic Medical Institute of Virginia," 288–89.

21. "The Scientific and Eclectic Medical Institute," *Western Medical Reformer* 7 (1847): 47–48; James O. Breeden, "Thomsonianism in Virginia," *Virginia Magazine of History and Biography* 82 (1974): 177.

22. Horatio C. Newton, "Death of Professor Calvin Newton, M.D.," *Worcester Journal of Medicine* 8 (1853): 290.

23. Newton, "Death of Professor Calvin Newton, M.D.," 291–92.

24. Galei, "History of Medical Reform in New England," *New England Botanic Medical and Surgical Journal* 5 (1851): 12–13; Calvin Newton, "Our Principles," *New England Botanic Medical and Surgical Journal* 5 (1851): 27.

25. Circular, "New England Botanico-Medical College," *New England Botanic Medical and Surgical Journal* 1 (1847): 23; Circular, "Annual Announcement," *New England Botanic Medical and Surgical Journal* 1 (1847): 325–26; Circular, "Announcement and Circular," *Worcester Journal of Medicine* 7 (1852): 317–23.

26. Newton, "Death of Professor Calvin Newton, M.D.," 292; Galei, "History of Medical Reform in New England," 13–14; I. M. Comings, "Explanation," *New England Botanic Medical and Surgical Journal* 1 (1847): 98–99.

27. "Worcester Botanico-Medical College," *New England Botanic Medical and Surgical Journal* 1 (1847): 317–19.

28. "Proposed Courtesy of the Medical Institute of Virginia," *New England Botanic Medical and Surgical Journal* 1 (1847): 277–78.

29. "Professional Courtesy," *New England Botanic Medical and Surgical Journal* 1 (1847): 291.

30. "New England Botanico-Medical College," *New England Botanic Medical and Surgical Journal* 2 (1848): 53.

31. Palemon John, "The Name Question," in *The American Journal of Medical Reform, for the People and the Profession*, ed. J. D. Friend and H. M. Sweet (New York: H. Winchester, 1857), 252–53.

32. "Medical Reform," in Friend and Sweet, *The American Journal of Medical Reform, for the People and the Profession*, 244–45.

33. John Kost, "Letter to the Reformed Medical Convention," in Friend and Sweet, *The American Journal of Medical Reform, for the People and the Profession*, 183.

34. Galei, "History of Medical Reform in New England," 16.

35. Alva Curtis, "Letter from Dr. Curtis to Calvin Newton," *New England Botanic Medical and Surgical Journal* 2 (1848): 341.

36. Calvin Newton, "Botanico-Medical College of Ohio, Cincinnati," *New England Botanic Medical and Surgical Journal* 2 (1848): 272.

37. Galei, "History of Medical Reform in New England," 14–15.

38. Ibid., 18; Newton, "Death of Professor Calvin Newton, M.D.," 293.

39. Galei, "History of Medical Reform in New England," 20.

40. Ibid., 23.

41. "The Clinic's Home," *Worcester Journal of Medicine* 7 (1852): 322–23.

42. "Botanico-Medical College," *New England Botanic Medical and Surgical Journal* 1 (1847): 114–15.

43. Editorial, "Our Next College Class," *New England Botanic Medical and Surgical Journal* 5 (1851): 351, 355; Circular, "Announcement and Circular," *Worcester Journal of Medicine* 7 (1852): 320.

44. Circular, "Announcement and Circular," 318.

45. E. M. Parritt, "Worcester Medical Institution; Meeting of Its Trustees," *New England Botanic Medical and Surgical Journal* 3 (1849), 353; Editor, "Our Next College Class," *New England Botanic Medical and Surgical Journal* 5 (1851): 351. The hydropaths, or what remained of the sect, did not fully endorse physio-medicalism until 1891. See J. H. Hanaford, "The Treatment of Disease," *Phrenological Journal* 90 (1891): 105.

46. Circular, "Announcement and Circular," 318.

47. Editorial, "Our Next College Class," *New England Botanic Medical and Surgical Journal* 5 (1851): 350–56.

48. Ibid., 353.

49. Circular, "Announcement and Circular," 319.

50. Galei, "History of Medical Reform in New England," 19–20.

51. Ibid., 21. After leaving the college, and following the death of Newton, Isaac M. Comings continued his feud with Frank H. Kelley, the new editor of the *Worcester Journal of Medicine*. Comings also made an unsuccessful bid to establish a rival college. See Editor, "The Worcester Medical College and Its Traducers," *Worcester Journal of Medicine* 9 (1854): 348–56.

52. Calvin Newton, "Address to Medical Eclectics Throughout the United States," *Worcester Journal of Medicine* 7 (1852): 285–86.

53. Calvin Newton, "Free Schools," *Worcester Journal of Medicine* 7 (1852): 321–22.

54. Calvin Newton, "I and U," *New England Botanic Medical and Surgical Journal* 2 (1848): 238.

55. Calvin Newton, "Worcester Medical Institution," *Worcester Journal of Medicine* 8 (1853): 35.

56. Calvin Newton, "Dr. Beach's School," *Worcester Journal of Medicine* 8 (1853): 134–35.

57. Newton, "Death of Professor Calvin Newton, M.D.," 293.

58. Trustees, "Address to the Friends of Medical Reform in New England," *Worcester Journal of Medicine* 8 (1853): 299.

59. L. Reuben, "An Address on the Life, Character, and Labors of the Late Professor Calvin Newton; Delivered Before the National Eclectic Medical Association, May 10th, 1854," *Worcester Journal of Medicine* 9 (1854): 182–94.

60. Editor, "Prize Essay," *Worcester Journal of Medicine* 9 (1854): 291; L. C. Dolley, "The Fundamental and Distinctive Principles of the Eclectic Practice of Medicine," *Worcester Journal of Medicine* 9 (1854): 299–326.

61. John King, "Concentrated Medicines Adulterated," *Worcester Journal of Medicine* 10 (1855): 225–27.

62. Edwin S. Wayne, "Examination of the Preparations Made by the American Chemical Institute, New York," *American Journal of Pharmacy* 27 (1855): 388; Scudder,

quoted in John Uri Lloyd, *The Eclectic Alkaloids, Resins, Resinoids, Oleo-Resins and Concentrated Principles* (Cincinnati: J. U. and C. G. Lloyd, 1910), 39.

63. Anthony, "Physio-Medicalism and Progress," 229.

64. "Charter of the Metropolitan Medical College," in Friend and Sweet, *American Journal of Medical Reform, for the People and the Profession*, 361; "Circular of the Metropolitan Medical College," in Friend and Sweet, *American Journal of Medical Reform, for the People and the Profession*, 366.

65. "Circular of the Metropolitan Medical College," 365–66.

66. "Joseph D. Friend," *Physio-Medical Journal* 16 (1890): 90–92.

67. W. H. Cook, "Higher Education," *Sanative Medicine* 4 (1894): 495; H. E. Firth, "The Origin of the American Eclectic Practice of Medicine, and Its Early History in the State of New York," *Transactions of the Eclectic Medical Society* 10 (1878): 202–3.

68. "Medical Reform," in Friend and Sweet, *The American Journal of Medical Reform, for the People and the Profession*, 247.

69. Berman, "Neo-Thomsonianism in the United States," 137–38.

70. B. A. Wright, "How to Advance Physio-Medicalism," *Physio-Medical Journal* 18 (1892): 239.

4. Years of Consolidation

1. Leslie B. Arey, "The Origin of the Graded Medical Curriculum," *Journal of Medical Education* 51 (1976): 1010–11; Martin Kaufman, *American Medical Education: The Formative Years, 1765–1910* (Westport, Conn.: Greenwood, 1976), 127–28; Thomas N. Bonner, *Medicine in Chicago, A Chapter in the Social and Scientific Development of a City, 1850–1950* (Madison: American History Research Center, 1957), 47–68.

2. Lester S. King, "The Painfully Slow Progress in Medical Education," *Journal of the American Medical Association* 249 (1983): 270–71; Craig F. Donatucci, "In Anticipation of Flexner," *Transactions and Studies, College of Physicians of Philadelphia*, Ser. 4, 44 (1978): 280–89.

3. Brookes Peters, "The Medical Student of the Late Nineteenth Century," *North Carolina Medical Journal* 40 (1979): 415–22; Lester S. King, "Medicine Seeks to be 'Scientific,'" *Journal of the American Medical Association* 249 (1983): 2475–79.

4. The eclectic Wooster Beach had been the family physician to William H. Cook when he was a boy. See William H. Cook, "Eclecticism," *Physio-Medical Recorder* 30 (1866): 133–50.

5. William H. Cook, "Medical Reform Associations," in *The American Journal of Medical Reform, for the People and the Profession*, ed. J. D. Friend and H. M. Sweet (New York: H. Winchester, 1857), 105–8.

6. "The Physio-Medical Institute," *Physio-Medical Recorder* 26 (1862): 84.

7. "Postponement of Lectures," *Physio-Medical Recorder* 26 (1862): 165.

8. "Physio-Medicalism in the Army," *Physio-Medical Recorder* 26 (1862): 104.

9. William H. Cook, "A Small Wedge," *Physio-Medical Recorder* 26 (1862): 165.

10. William H. Cook, "Thoughts for a President," *Physio-Medical Recorder* 26 (1862): 117–18.

11. Ibid., 121–23.

12. Hammond's Circular No. 6, in U.S. Government, Surgeon General's Office, *The Medical and Surgical History of the War of Rebellion* (1861–65). *Prepared in Accordance With the Acts of Congress, Under the Direction of Surgeon General Joseph K. Barnes, United States Army,* vol. 1, pt. 2 (Washington, D.C.: Government Printing Office, 1870–88), 719.

13. Quoted in "Communication," *Chicago Medical Journal and Examiner* 6 (1863): 321. See also "Calomel and Tartar Emetic in the Army," *American Medical Times* 6 (1863): 297; "Calomel and Tartar Emetic," *Medical and Surgical Reporter* 10 (1863): 275; "Calomel and Tartar Emetic as Remedial Agents," *Buffalo Medical and Surgical Journal* 3 (1863): 32.

14. J. F. Hibberd, "Circular No. 6 and the Profession," *Cincinnati Lancet and Observer* 6 (1863): 429; "Proceedings," *Transactions of the American Medical Association* 14 (1864): 23–34.

15. "The Death-Knell of Calomel," *Physio-Medical Recorder* 28 (1864): 89–90.

16. Circular, "Fifth Annual Announcement of the Physio-Medical Institute," *Physio-Medical Recorder* 28 (1864): 132; D. M. Marsh, "Physio-Medical Institute," *Physio-Medical Recorder* 31 (1867): 265–68.

17. William H. Cook, "The Cincinnati Hospital," *Physio-Medical Recorder* 35 (1871): 36–37, 382–86. See also John Harley Warner, *The Therapeutic Perspective; Medical Practice, Knowledge, and Identity in America, 1820–1885* (Cambridge: Harvard University Press, 1986), 115–61.

18. Cook, "The Cincinnati Hospital," 38, 384–85; Advertisement, "Drs. W. H. Cook and W. W. Cook," *Cincinnati Medical Gazette and Recorder* 52 (1884): 24.

19. Circular, "Physio-Medical Institute, Session of 1875–76," *Physio-Medical Recorder* 39 (1875): 131–38.

20. Illinois State Board of Health, "Report of the Illinois State Board of Health on Medical Education and the Regulation of the Practice of Medicine in the United States and Canada," *Journal of the American Medical Association* 22 (1894): 393. William H. Cook, "Diplomas of the Physio-Medical Institute," *Cincinnati Medical Gazette: A Journal of Medical Reform* 1 (1877): 350–51. The Illinois board passed a resolution in 1877 placing all medical colleges on notice that it would no longer recognize colleges that held two sessions in a single year, managing to graduate an individual after only seven months of study.

21. Illinois State Board of Health, "Report," 393. See also J. E. Emerson, "The Requirements for Preliminary Education in the Medical Colleges of the United States and Canada," *Journal of the American Medical Association* 14 (1890): 271–72. These recommendations became mandatory when the board announced that, after the 1882–83 sessions, it would recognize no college in "good standing" that did not conform to the requirements.

22. Cook, "Diplomas of the Physio-Medical Institute," 350–51.

23. William H. Cook, "Diplomas Honorable and Dishonorable," *Cincinnati Medical Gazette: A Journal of Medical Reform* 1 (1877): 166.

24. Alumnus, "Medical Colleges and Education," *Cincinnati Medical Gazette: A Journal of Medical Reform* 1 (1877): 370–71.

25. William H. Cook, "Higher Education," *Sanative Medicine* 4 (1894): 496; William H. Cook, "Buchanan and His Bogus Diplomas," *Cincinnati Medical Gazette and Recorder* 44 (1880): 306–7.

26. Letter quoted in William H. Cook, "Shall It be Honor or Dishonor?" *Cincinnati Medical Gazette and Recorder* 45 (1881): 130. See also letter from Gideon Lincecum to H. H. Hill (botanic pharmacist) of Cincinnati, January 1, 1866, in Gideon Lincecum,

Lincecum Papers, Letterpress, 1865–67 (Austin: Barker Texas History Center, University of Texas).

27. Cook, "Shall It be Honor or Dishonor?" 131.

28. William H. Cook, "Medical Legislation," *Cincinnati Medical Gazette and Recorder* 44 (1880), 324.

29. William H. Cook, "A Champion of Corruption," *Cincinnati Medical Gazette and Recorder* 55 (1881): 64.

30. Editor, "Diplomas and Professorships Wanted," *Cincinnati Medical Gazette and Recorder* 45 (1881), 34–35.

31. Quoted in William H. Cook, "A Diploma for Everybody," *Physio-Medical Recorder* 26 (1862): 169.

32. William H. Cook, "Diplomas and Medical Laws," *Cincinnati Medical Gazette: A Journal of Medical Reform* 1 (1877): 261.

33. Ibid., 263.

34. Ibid.

35. Anthony, "Physio-Medicalism and Progress," *Physio-Medical Journal* 12 (1886): 234.

36. William H. Cook, "Financial Policy of the P.-M. Institute," *Physio-Medical Recorder* 36 (1872): 529, 547–49.

37. Ibid., 529.

38. William H. Cook, "Education in the Physio-Medical Institute," *Physio-Medical Recorder* 37 (1873): 557.

39. Ibid., 558.

40. Anthony, "Physio-Medicalism and Progress," 231.

41. Editor, "Death Claims the Best Known Physiomedicalist in the Country," *Physio-Medical Record* 9 (1906): 1–2.

42. George Hasty, "Andrew Wallace," *Physio-Medical Journal*, 19 (1893): 37–40.

43. "G. N. Davidson," *Physio-Medical Journal* 19 (1893): 348–50; Alexander Wilder, "Outline History of Eclectic Medicine," *Transactions of the National Eclectic Medical Association* 5 (1877): 44–45.

44. "In Memoriam," *Physio-Medical Journal* 8 (1882): 218–19.

45. "College Commencement," *Physio-Medical Journal* 13 (1887): 126; 15 (1889): 27–28; 15 (1890), 287; W. F. Stouder, "Our Class," *Physio-Medical Journal* 14 (1888): 112.

46. "The College," *Physio-Medical Journal* 16 (1890): 125.

47. "College Commencement," *Physio-Medical Journal* 18 (1892): 143.

48. *Nineteenth Annual Announcement of the Physio-Medical College of Indiana* (Indianapolis: Baker-Randolph, 1891), 6–8, 19–20.

49. Ibid., 21–22.

50. Ibid., 22.

51. Ibid., 27–28.

52. "New Free Dispensary," *Sanative Medicine* 4 (1894): 97.

53. "P-M Dispensary," *Physio-Medical Journal* 20 (1894): 408–9.

54. Ibid., 410.

55. "Medical Schools in the United States," *Journal of the American Medical Association* 37 (1901): 747; Advertisement, *Physio-Medical Record* 8 (March 1905): back page.

56. Advertisement, *Physio-Medical Record* 8 (March 1905): back page; "Medical Schools in the United States (1904)," *Journal of the American Medical Association* 43 (1904): 491.

57. "Sanative Medicine in England," *Physio-Medical Record* 7 (1904): 67–68.

58. E. Grove Anthony, "A New Order of Things at the Physio-Medical College of Indiana," *Physio-Medical Record* 9 (1906): 165–67.

59. Editor, "A Plea for Justice," *Physio-Medical Record* 10 (1907): 132–33.

60. Editor, "A Plea for Justice," 134, 136.

61. Editor, "A Business Manager," *Physio-Medical Record* 9 (1906): 15.

62. Nathan D. Woodard, "The Indiana State Sanitarium," *Physio-Medical Record* 9 (1906): 167.

63. Editor, "Plans for a Hospital for the Physio-Medical College of Indiana," *Physio-Medical Record* 10 (1907): 213.

64. Editor, "A New National Society," *Physio-Medical Record* 10 (1907): 9; Burton D. Myers, *The History of Medical Education in Indiana* (Bloomington: University of Indiana Press, 1956), 78; J. H. Brayton, "The Development of Medical Education in Indiana" (master's thesis, Indiana University, 1929), 52.

65. Correspondence with Martha E. Wright, Reference Librarian, Indiana State Library; M. Virginia Dwyer, ed., *American Medical Directory*, 20th ed. (Chicago: American Medical Association, 1958), 38; Brayton, "The Development of Medical Education in Indiana," 48–52; Max R. Hyman, *Journal Handbook of Indianapolis* (Indianapolis: Indianapolis Journal Newspaper Company, 1902), 224.

66. Dwyer, *American Medical Directory*, 43, 44.

67. J. B. Jacques, "Thoughts of a Layman," *Physio-Medical Journal* 19 (1893): 98; M. Veenboer, "Physio-Medical Physician," *Physio-Medical Journal* 14 (1888): 109.

68. J. W. Neel, "Sanative Versus Natural Medication," *Physio-Medical Journal* 18 (1892): 431.

69. G. N. Davidson, "Annual Address," *Physio-Medical Journal* 9 (1883): 201; Jacques, "Thoughts of a Layman," 98.

5. Vitalism and the Materia Medica

1. Charles E. Woodruff, "Modern Vitalism," *New York Medical Journal* 94 (1911): 361. See also R. C. Bond, "Vitalism and Vital Medication," *Cincinnati Lancet and Observer* 20 (1877): 446; Joseph O'Carroll, "Vitalism in the Practice of Medicine," *Dublin Journal of Medical Sciences* 134 (1912): 404–5.

2. S. J. Melzer, "Vitalism and Mechanism in Biology and Medicine," *Science* 19 (1904): 20.

3. Quoted in Charles S. Myers, "Vitalism: A Brief Historical and Critical Review," *Mind* (1900): 227; Norman Kemp Smith, *New Studies in the Philosophy of Descartes* (London: Macmillan, 1952); Thomas S. Kuhn, "Descartes: Physiological Methods," *Journal of the History of Biology* 3 (1970): 53–79.

4. J. M. Thurston, "The Problem of Life," *Physio-Medical Journal* 11 (1885): 110.

5. Melville C. Keith, *Keith's Domestic Practice and Botanic Hand Book* (Bellville, Ohio: Published by Author, 1901), 49–69.

6. Alva Curtis, *A Fair Examination and Criticism of All the Medical Systems in Vogue* (Cincinnati: Printed for the Proprietor, 1865), 194.

7. H. J. Treat, "Disease—What Is It?" *Physio-Medical Record* 9 (1906): 199–200.

8. Thurston, "The Problem of Life," 97.

9. J. M. Thurston, "Medical Sectarianism a Necessity to Progress—Usurpation of Political Power and Governmental Patronage Wrong in any Sect—Equal Rights and Justice to All Schools as Guaranteed," *Physio-Medical Record* 7 (1904): 206.

10. Burton D. Myers, *The History of Medical Education in Indiana* (Bloomington: University of Indiana Press, 1956), 78.

11. Quoted in Editor, "The Indiana Physio-Medical Association," *Physio-Medical Record* 9 (1906): 110.

12. Ibid., 111.

13. C. A. Stafford, "The Breadth and Advanced Ideas Contained in a Medical Education," *Physio-Medical Journal* 20 (1894): 367.

14. Ibid., 369.

15. J. S. Byers, "Some Thoughts on Vitality," *Physio-Medical Journal* 13 (1887): 291.

16. Ibid., 233.

17. J. Redding, "That Vitality Question," *Physio-Medical Journal* 13 (1887): 241.

18. George Hasty, "That Discussion. Needless Alarm," *Physio-Medical Journal* 8 (1882): 384.

19. Editor, "Proceedings of the American Association of Physio-Medical Physicians and Surgeons," *Physio-Medical Journal* 15 (1890): 359.

20. G. N. Davidson, "Fundamental Principles," *Physio-Medical Journal* 15 (1889): 20.

21. Joseph M. Thurston, *The Philosophy of Physiomedicalism. Its Theorem, Corollary, and Laws of Application for the Cure of Disease* (Richmond, Ind.: Nicholson Printing and Manufacturing, 1900), 317, 324.

22. William R. Dunham, *Theory of Medical Science. The Doctrine of an Inherent Power in Medicine a Fallacy: The Ultimate Special Properties of Vitality and the Laws of Vital Force Constitute the Fundamental Basis of Medical Philosophy and Science* (Boston: James Campbell, 1876), 6, 82, 99.

23. Thurston, *Philosophy of Physiomedicalism*, 218.

24. Ibid., 366.

25. Ibid., 252–53, 255–56.

26. J. Ben Nichols, "Physio-Medicalism," *Medical News* 66 (1895): 153.

27. Elder A. W. Bartlett, "Increase of Knowledge in Medical Science," *Physio-Medical Journal* 19 (1893): 117.

28. William H. Cook, *The Physio-Medical Dispensatory: A Treatise on Therapeutics, Materia Medica, and Pharmacy, in Accordance with the Principles of Physiological Medication* (Cincinnati: By Author, 1869), 7.

29. F. O. Broady, "A Medical Practice Without Alcohol and Without Poisons," *Physio-Medical Record* 6 (1903): 261.

30. Advertisements, *New England Botanic Medical and Surgical Journal* 1 (1847): 118–20; Alex Berman, "The Thomsonian Movement and Its Relation to American Pharmacy and Medicine," *Bulletin of the History of Medicine* 25 (1951): 521–22.

31. "What of Drugs," *Physio-Medical Journal* 10 (1884): 130; "The Physio-Medical Drug House," *Sanative Medicine* 4 (1894): 73; Melville C. Keith, "The Remedies We Use," *Physio-Medical Journal* 13 (1887): 146.

32. "Eli Lilly and Co.," *Physio-Medical Journal*, 16 (1890): 126.

33. "The Great Pill Maker," *Physio-Medical Journal* 7 (1881): 61.

34. Keith, "The Remedies We Use," 146.

35. Horton Howard, *An Improved System of Botanic Medicine Founded Upon Correct Physiological Principles, Comprising a Complete Treatise on the Practice of Medicine* (Cincinnati: Kost, Bigger and Hart, 1832), 409–11; T. J. Lyle, *Physio-Medical Therapeutics, Materia Medica, and Pharmacy* (Salem, Ohio: J. M. Lyle and Brothers, 1897), 58–59.

36. John Albert Burnett, "A Selection of Thirty Physio-Medical Remedies," *Physio-Medical Record* 9 (1906): 124.

37. Alex Berman, "Neo-Thomsonianism in the United States," *Journal of the History of Medicine* 10 (1956): 149.

38. N. E. Harold, "The Best Physiomedical Tonic," *Physio-Medical Record* 8 (1905): 123–25.

39. Howard, *An Improved System of Botanic Medicine Founded Upon Correct Physiological Principles*, 413–60.

40. Thurston, *Philosophy of Physiomedicalism*, 97–98, 102.

41. A. H. Baird, "Phthisis Pulmonalis," *Physio-Medical Journal* 16 (1890): 33–35, 38–39, 41–42; Editor, "American Association of Physio-Medical Physicians and Surgeons—Eleventh Annual Session," *Physio-Medical Journal* 19 (1893): 209; Melville C. Keith, *Childbirth and the Child: A Treatise for Parents and Nurses on the Care of the Mother and Child, During Gestation, Pregnancy and Parturition* (Minneapolis: Alfred Roper, 1888), 120–21.

42. Baird, "Phthisis Pulmonalis," 33–35, 38–39, 41–42; Editor, "American Association of Physio-Medical Physicians and Surgeons—Eleventh Annual Session," 209; Keith, *Childbirth and the Child*, 120–21.

43. Alva Curtis, *The Provocation and the Reply: Or, Allopathy Versus Physio-Medicalism in a Review of Prof. M. B. Wright's Remarks at the Dedication of the Cincinnati New Hospital, January 8th, 1869* (Cincinnati: Published for the Proprietor, 1870), 38.

44. A. H. Baird, "Alcohol," *Physio-Medical Journal* 8 (1882): 310–11.

45. Editor, "Tobacco—Coffee—Tea," *Oregon Physio-Medical Journal* 2 (1868): 231.

46. Keith, *Childbirth and the Child*, 11.

47. G. H. Mayhugh, "In Memorium," *Sanative Medicine* 1 (1892): 214.

48. Manasseh Cutler, "An Account of Some of the Vegetable Productions Naturally Growing in This Part of America, Botanically Arranged," *Memoirs of the Academy of the Arts and Sciences* 1 (1785): 396–493. John Uri Lloyd, *Origin and History of All the Pharmacopeial Vegetable Drugs, Chemicals and Preparations* (Cincinnati: Caxton Press, 1921), 184; Leaman F. Hallett, "Medicine and Pharmacy of the New England Indians," *Bulletin of the Massachusetts Archaeological Society* 17 (1955): 46–49; H. W. Youngken, "Drugs of the North American Indians," *American Journal of Pharmacy* 96 (1925): 485–502.

49. William H. Cook, *The Physio-Medical Dispensatory*, 519–21.

50. Ibid., 543–49.

51. Nichols, "Physio-Medicalism," 154.

52. J. Simmons, "Is Lobelia a Poison?" *Physio-Medical Journal* 19 (1893): 40–41.

53. Robert A Buerki, "The Reception of the Germ Theory of Disease in the American Journal of Pharmacy," *Pharmacy in History* 13 (1971): 158–68; H. A. Lechevalier and M. Solotorovsky, *Three Centuries of Microbiology* (New York: McGraw Hill, 1965); J. K. Crellin, "The Dawn of Germ Theory: Particles, Infection, and Biology," in F. N. L. Poynter, *Medicine and Science in the 1860s: Proceedings of the 6th British Congress on the History of Medicine* (London: Welcome Institute for the History of Medicine, 1968), 57–76; William Bulloch, *The History of Bacteriology* (London: Oxford University Press, 1938).

54. George Hasty, "New Cures," *Physio-Medical Journal* 20 (1894): 428–30.

55. Roger T. Farley, "Physio-Medical Antitoxin," *Physio-Medical Record* 5 (1902): 152.

56. Thurston, *The Philosophy of Physiomedicalism*, 299–300.

57. Farley, "Physio-Medical Antitoxin," 155.

58. George Hasty, "Phthisis Pulmonalis," *Physio-Medical Journal* 18 (1892): 125–28.

59. Thurston, *The Philosophy of Physiomedicalism*, 302.

60. Editor, "Proceedings of the Thirty-Third Annual Session of the Indiana Physio-Medical Association," *Physio-Medical Journal* 21 (1895): 160–62.

61. Quoted in Editor, "Proceedings of the Thirty-Third Annual Session of the Indiana Physio-Medical Association," 163.

62. Thurston, *The Philosophy of Physiomedicalism*, 303.

63. F. O. Broady, "Are Bacteria Pathogenic?" *Sanative Medicine* 4 (1894): 125–38.

64. Thomson quoted in Hermance, "The Germ Theory of Disease—Is It True or False?" *Physio-Medical Journal* 21 (1895): 94, 97, 100–101.

65. Hermance, "The Germ Theory of Disease—Is It True or False?" 104.

66. Editorial, "At It Again," *Physio-Medical Journal* 8 (1882): 253–54.

67. "The Bacteriological Craze," *Sanative Medicine* 4 (1894): 167.

68. "The Microbe Causation Theory," *Sanative Medicine* 14 (1904): 8.

69. Thurston, *Philosophy of Physiomedicalism*, 8–9.

70. Cited in Berman, "Neo-Thomsonianism in the United States," 150.

71. J. C. Shelton, "Application of the Fundamental Principles of Medical Science to Clinical Practice," *Oregon Physio-Medical Journal* 1 (1866): 100–101.

6. "The American"

1. Donald E. Konold, *A History of American Medical Ethics, 1847–1912* (Madison: University of Wisconsin Press, 1962); Joseph F. Kett, *The Formation of the American Medical Profession: The Role of Institutions, 1780–1860* (New Haven: Yale University Press, 1968), 165–77; John S. Haller, Jr., *Medical Protestants: The Eclectics in American Medicine, 1825–1939* (Carbondale: Southern Illinois University Press, 1993), 55–56.

2. Editor, "Miscellaneous," *Western Medical Reformer* 2 (1837): 334.

3. Editor, "The National P.-M. Convention of 1852," *Cincinnati Medical Gazette and Recorder* 44 (1880): 292.

4. Ibid., 293–94.

5. Alva Curtis, *A Fair Examination and Criticism of All the Medical Systems in Vogue*, 2nd ed. (Cincinnati: Printed for the Proprietor, 1865), 188–89.

6. E. Anthony, "Physio-Medicalism and Progress," *Physio-Medical Recorder* 12 (1886): 230–31.

7. Editor, "The National P.-M. Convention of 1852," 294–95.

8. Alex Berman, "Neo-Thomsonianism in the United States," *Journal of the History of Medicine* 2 (1956): 135–36.

9. Editor, "A National Convention," *Cincinnati Medical Gazette and Recorder* 44 (1880): 38.

10. William H. Cook and H. E. Hoke, "A National P.-M. Convention," *Cincinnati Medical Gazette and Recorder* 44 (1880): 184.

11. Ibid., 186.

12. Quoted in Cook and Hoke, "A National P.-M. Convention," 186.

13. Cook and Hoke, "A National P.-M. Convention," 188.

14. Quoted in Cook and Hoke, "A National P.-M. Convention," 189.

15. Cook and Hoke, "A National P.-M. Convention," 185.

16. William H. Cook, "About a National P.-M. Convention," *Cincinnati Gazette and Recorder* 44 (1880): 234, 236–37.

17. Cook, "About a National P.-M. Convention," 250.

18. Ibid.

19. A.H. Baird, "National Convention," *Physio-Medical Journal* 7 (1881): 19–20.

20. William H. Cook, "Notes and Queries," *Physio-Medical Journal* 9 (1883): 158.

21. Cook, "Notes and Queries," 158.

22. Editor, "A National Physio-Medical Association," *Physio-Medical Journal* 9 (1883): 94.

23. William Wesley Cook, "American Physio-Medical Convention," *Cincinnati Medical Gazette and Recorder* 51 (1883): 98.

24. Berman, "Neo-Thomsonianism in the United States," 139.

25. Editor, "Proceedings of the National Convention," *Physio-Medical Journal* 11 (1883): 163–64.

26. Editor, "Proceedings of the National Convention," 165.

27. William H. Cook, "The National Convention," *Cincinnati Medical Gazette and Recorder* 51 (1883): 87.

28. Editorial, "The National Convention," *Physio-Medical Journal* 9 (1883): 188–89.

29. William Wesley Cook, "Official Report, Transactions of the Second Annual Convention of the American Association of Physio-Medical Physicians and Surgeons, Cincinnati, May, 1884," *Healthside* 52 (1884): 25. William Wesley Cook was secretary of the convention.

30. Cook, "Official Report," 26.

31. Editorial, "The Germ Theory," *Healthside* 52 (1884): 45.

32. Cook, "Official Report," 28.

33. Ibid., 28–29.

34. Ibid., 29.

35. Ibid., 31.

36. George Hasty, "The American," *Physio-Medical Recorder* 10 (1884): 198. William Wesley Cook, who attended eye and ear cases, shared a practice in Cincinnati with William H. Cook, who specialized in nervous disorders and diseases of women.

37. William H. Cook, "Organize Societies," *Cincinnati Medical Gazette and Recorder* 52 (1884): 19.

38. Quoted in D.H. Stafford, "American Association of Physio-Medical Physicians and Surgeons, Third Annual Session," *Physio-Medical Journal* 11 (1885): 165–66.

39. Letter from William H. Cook to A.F. Elliot, April 17, 1885, in Editor, "American Association of Physio-Medical Physicians and Surgeons," *Physio-Medical Journal* 11 (1885): 166.

40. Letter of William Wesley Cook to William H. Cook, June 3, 1884, in Editor, "American Association of Physio-Medical Physicians and Surgeons," 167.

41. Ibid., 170.

42. Ibid., 194.

43. Editor, "Proceedings of the American Association of Physio-Medical Physicians and Surgeons," *Physio-Medical Journal* 15 (1890): 359; "Indiana Physio-Medical Association; Twenty-Fourth Session," *Physio-Medical Journal* 12 (1886): 146–56.

44. Editor, "The National Association of Physio-Medical Physicians and Surgeons," *Physio-Medical Record* 6 (1903): 111–12.

45. Editor, "Twenty-Third Annual Session," *Physio-Medical Record* 8 (1905): 174.

46. Ibid., 185.

47. J.M. Thurston, "Cholera," *Physio-Medical Journal* 9 (1885): 21.

48. Joseph M. Thurston, *The Philosophy of Physiomedicalism. Its Theorem, Corollary, and Laws of Application for the Cure of Disease* (Richmond, Ind.: Nicholson Printing and Manufacturing, 1900), 367.

49. Editor, "A New National Society," *Physio-Medical Record* 10 (1907): 1.

50. Ibid., 3–4.

51. "An Ass in the Profession," *Physio-Medical Journal* 17 (1891): 406.

52. Quoted in J. Simmons, "Is Lobelia a Poison?" *Physio-Medical Journal* 19 (1893): 56.

53. Quoted in George Hasty "Relation of the Eclectic Board to Physio-Medicalism," *Physio-Medical Journal* 14 (1888): 241–42.

54. Quoted in ibid., 242.

55. Ibid., 243.

56. Ibid., 243.

57. A.A. Abernathy, "Medical Legislation," *Physio-Medical Journal* 17 (1891): 87–88.

58. Quoted in F. Vernette, "Lobelia a Poison," *Physio-Medical Journal* 19 (1893): 94–95.

59. Editorial, "Notes and Queries," *Physio-Medical Journal* 16 (1890): 26–28.

60. J. M. Thurston, "Medical Sectarianism a Necessity to Progress—Usurpation of Political Power and Governmental Patronage Wrong in Any Sect—Equal Rights and Justice to All Schools as Guaranteed," *Physio-Medical Record* 7 (1904): 205.

61. A.H. Baird, "Be Up and Doing," *Physio-Medical Journal* 17 (1891): 71–74.

62. Alexander Wilder, *History of Medicine: A Brief Outline of Medical History From the Earliest Historic Period With an Extended Account of the Various Sects of Physicians and New Schools of Medicine in Later Centuries* (Augusta, Maine: Maine Farmer Publishing, 1904), 883–84; John M. Scudder, "Let Them Go," *Eclectic Medical Journal* 56 (1896): 54–55.

63. Editor, "Notes and Queries," *Physio-Medical Journal* 16 (1890): 94.

64. Editor, "American Association of Physio-Medical Physicians and Surgeons—Ninth Session," *Physio-Medical Journal* 17 (1891): 177, 179.

65. Thurston, "Medical Sectarianism a Necessity to Progress," 202.

66. Editor, "State Associations," *Physio-Medical Journal* 12 (1886): 156.

67. Editor, "The Newest Physio-Medical Association," *Physio-Medical Record* 10 (1907): 116.

68. W.A. Spurgeon, "Letter from Doctor Spurgeon," *Physio-Medical Record* 8 (1905): 110.

69. "Statistics," *Eclectic Medical Journal* 54 (1894): 396.

70. J. Ben Nichols, "Physio-Medicalism," *Medical News* 65 (1895): 152.

71. Frederick C. Waite, "Sectarian Medicine in Ohio," *Ohio State Medical Journal* 49 (1953): 50. In 1938, there were fewer than 160 sectarians practicing in Ohio, or 1.75 percent of the total number of practicing physicians.

7. Final Years

1. "Medical Education in the United States (1914)," *Journal of the American Medical Association* 63 (1914): 685.

2. Ibid.

3. John Benjamin Nichols, "Medical Sectarianism," *Journal of the American Medical Association* 60 (1913): 335.

4. Ibid.

5. Arthur Dean Bevan, "Medical Education and the Hospital," *Journal of the American Medical Association* 60 (1913): 975.

6. Ibid.

7. Ibid., 978.

8. Ibid., 976.

9. Ibid.

10. Ibid., 977.

11. Quoted in Walter A. Wells, "Medical Education and the State," *Journal of the American Medical Association* 38 (1902): 863; John M. Dodson, "The Modern University School—Its Purposes and Methods," *Journal of the American Medical Association* 39 (1902): 521–29; William Osler, "The Natural Method of Teaching the Subject of Medicine," *Journal of the American Medical Association* 36 (1901): 1673–79.

12. Douglas Carroll, Jr., "The Contribution of the Johns Hopkins University School of Medicine," *Maryland State Medical Journal* 30 (1981): 76–78; A. McGehee Harvey, *Adventures in Medical Research: A Century of Discovery at Johns Hopkins* (Baltimore: Johns Hopkins University Press, 1976); A.M. Chesney, *The Johns Hopkins Hospital and the Johns Hopkins University School of Medicine*, 3 vols. (Baltimore: Johns Hopkins University Press, 1943, 1958, 1963); Eileen R. Cunningham, "A Short Review of the Development of Medical Education and Schools of Medicine," *Annals of Medical History* 7 (1935): 237–40; Douglas Hubble, "William Osler and Medical Education," *Journal of the Royal College of Physicians of London* 9 (1975): 269–78.

13. Henry S. Pritchett, "Medical Progress," *Journal of the American Medical Association* 60 (1913): 743–46.

14. Howard S. Berliner, "A Larger Perspective on the Flexner Report," *International Journal of Health Services* 5 (1975): 583–84; Abraham Flexner, *Medical Education in the United States and Canada; A Report to the Carnegie Foundation on the Advancement of Teaching* (New York: Carnegie Foundation, 1910), 158.

15. George H. Simmons, "Medical Education and Preliminary Requirements," *Journal of the American Medical Association* 42 (1904): 1207.

16. Quoted in Dean F. Smiley, "History of the Association of American Medical Colleges, 1876–1957," *Journal of Medical Education* 32 (1957): 518.

17. Ibid., 520.

18. Bevan, "Medical Education and Hospitals," 975.

19. Quoted in *Annual Announcement of the Chicago Physio-Medical College* (Chicago: William Johnston Printing, 1891), 6.

20. Editorial, "To Chicago," *Physio-Medical Journal* 9 (1885): 363–64.

21. George Hasty, "Relation of the Eclectic Board to Physio-Medicalism," *Physio-Medical Journal* 14 (1888): 244.

22. William H. Cook, "Higher Education," *Sanative Medicine* 3 (1894): 515.

23. *Annual Announcement of the Chicago Physio-Medical College*, 6; H. P. Nelson, "Read This," *Sanative Medicine* 14 (1904): 11.

24. J. E. Roop, "Chicago Physio Medical College," *Sanative Medicine* 8 (1898): 203; *Annual Announcement of the Chicago Physio-Medical College*, 4; Announcement, "Chicago Physio-Medical College," *Sanative Medicine* 6 (1896): n.p.

25. *Annual Announcement of the Chicago Physio-Medical College*, 7, 21–22.

26. Ibid., 8, 17.

27. W. F. Pechuman, "Our Chicago College," *Sanative Medicine* 5 (1895): 121.

28. *Annual Announcement of the Chicago Physio-Medical College*, 17–18.

29. "A New Physio-Medical College," *Sanative Medicine* 7 (1897): 214.

30. A. E. Gammage, "Chicago College of Medicine and Surgery," *Sanative Medicine* 10 (1900): 140–41; "Medical Schools of the United States (1901)," *Journal of the American Medical Association* 37 (1901): 747.

31. "Medical Schools in the United States (1904)," *Journal of the American Medical Association* 42 (1904): 491.

32. P. Holt, "Texas Physio Medical Association," *Physio-Medical Journal* 10 (1884): 204–11.

33. J. M. Massie, "Report from Texas," *Physio-Medical Record* 9 (1906): 237–39.

34. Editor, "From Texas Students," *Physio-Medical Record* 8 (1905): 35–36; Advertisement, "Physiomedical College of Texas," *Sanative Medicine* 13 (1903): n.p.; "Medical Schools in the United States," *Journal of the American Medical Association* 39 (1902): 566.

35. F. O. Broady, "A Last Call," *Sanative Medicine* 4 (1895): 249.

36. Editor, "Our Colleges," *Physio-Medical Record* 10 (1907): 190–91; Massie, "Report from Texas," 239.

37. L. H. Painter, "Letter to the Editor," *Physio-Medical Record* 10 (1907): 167.

38. Flexner, *Medical Education in the United States and Canada*, 213

39. Flexner, *Medical Education in the United States and Canada*, 216–18, 220.

40. "State Board Statistics for 1911," *Journal of the American Medical Association* 58 (1911): 1599.

41. Alex Berman, "Neo-Thomsonianism in the United States," *Journal of the History of Medicine* 10 (1956): 142.

42. W. A. Harris, "Queries," *Physio-Medical Journal* 16 (1890): 86–87.

43. Berman, "Neo-Thomsonianism in the United States," 147.

44. A good example of this is Florence Dressler's *Feminology: A Guide for Womankind, Giving in Detail Instructions as to Motherhood, Maidenhood, and the Nursery* (Chicago: C. L. Dressler and Company, 1902), which relied on the eclectic works of William Byrd Powell, Joseph Rodes Buchanan, and Edward B. Foote; opposition of medicines that were mineral-based; and reliance on simple herbal recipes for sickness and hygiene. Dressler was a physician, faculty member, and secretary of the College of Medicine and Surgery (Physio-Medical) of Chicago.

45. John W. Shockey, "The History of Physio-Medicalism," *Physio-Medical Record* 9 (1906): 175–76.

46. Ibid., 179.

47. E. M. Haggard, "President's Address," *Physio-Medical Record* 9 (1906): 233.

48. Simmons, "Medical Education and Preliminary Requirements," 1206.

49. William G. Rothstein, *American Physicians in the Nineteenth Century: From Sects to Science* (Baltimore: Johns Hopkins University Press, 1972), 166, 228, 238–39.

50. John S. Haller, Jr., *Medical Protestants: The Eclectics in American Medicine, 1825–1939* (Carbondale: Southern Illinois University Press, 1993), chapter four.

51. Calvin Newton, "Our Medical Philosophy," *Worcester Journal of Medicine* 9 (1854): 289.

52. Quoted in "Periscope: Biographical Sketches," *Eclectic Medical Journal* 90 (1930): 184.

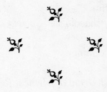

Selected Bibliography

This book has been researched chiefly from books, pamphlets, and journal articles. To assist the interested reader, I have included a complete listing of books and pamphlets used, as well as of certain general works that afford insight into the period and the subject as a whole, and I have listed all journals cited in the text and notes.

Journals Cited in Text

American Journal of Medical Reform, for the People and the Profession
American Journal of Pharmacy
American Journal of Science and Arts
American Medical Times
American Medicine
Annals of Medical History
Annals of the New York Academy of Sciences
Archiv fur Geschichte der Philosophie
Badger Pharmacist
Bedrock
Boston Medical and Surgical Journal
Botanic Record and Family Herbal

Botanico-Medical Recorder
British Journal of the History of Science
Buffalo Medical and Surgical Journal
Bulletin of the History of Medicine
Bulletin of the Massachusetts Archaeological Society
California Medical Journal
Chicago Medical Journal and Examiner
Cincinnati Lancet and Observer
Cincinnati Medical Gazette: A Journal of Medical Reform
Cincinnati Medical Gazette and Recorder
Coffin's Botanical Journal and Medical Reformer
College and Clinical Record
Colorado Medical Journal
Dublin Journal of Medical Sciences
Eclectic, and Medical Botanist (The)
Eclectic Medical Journal
Guy's Hospital Gazette
Healthside, A Monthly Journal Devoted to the Interests of Sound Bodies and Long
    Life
Indiana Journal of Medicine
International Journal of Health Services
Isis
Journal of the American Association of Physio-Medical Physicians and Surgeons
Journal of the American Institute of Homeopathy
Journal of the American Medical Association
Journal of the American Pharmaceutical Association
Journal of Health Conducted by the Physicians of the Cincinnati Dispensary and
    Vaccine Institution
Journal of Health and Practical Education
Journal of the History of Biology
Journal of the History of Medicine
Journal of Homoeopathics
Journal of Medical Education
Journal of Medical Reform
Journal of the Medical Society of New Jersey
Journal of the Royal College of Physicians of London
Ladies' Health Journal
Maryland State Medical Journal
Medical Analetic
Medical and Surgical Reporter
Medical Faculty Bulletin, Tulane University
Medical History
Medical Journal of Reform

Medical News

Medical Reformer

Medical Standard

Medical Times and Gazette

Memoirs of the Academy of the Arts and Sciences

Mind

New England Botanic Medical and Surgical Journal

New England Journal of Medicine

New England Medical Eclectic and Guide to Health

New York Medical Journal

New York State Journal of Medicine

North Carolina Medical Journal

Ohio State Archaeological and Historical Quarterly

Ohio State Medical Journal

Oregon Physio-Medical Journal

Osiris

Pharmacy in History

Philosophical Review

Phrenological Journal

Phronesis

Physiologico-Medical Recorder and Surgical Journal

Physio-Medical Journal

Physio-Medical Record

Physio-Medical Recorder

Physio-Medical Recorder and Surgical Journal

Popular Science Monthly

Proceedings of the Philadelphia County Medical Society

Proceedings of the Royal Society of Medicine

Publications, Cambridge Historical Society

Sanative Medicine

Science

Science Progress in the Twentieth Century

Scientific Monthly

Southern Medical Journal

Southern Medical Reformer

Southern Practitioner

Studies in the History and Method of Science

Studies in the History and Philosophy of Science

Synthesis

Thomsonian Recorder

Transactions of the American Medical Association

Transactions of the Association of American Physicians

Transactions of the Eclectic Medical Society

Transactions of the Medical Association of Georgia
Transactions of the National Eclectic Medical Association
Transactions of the Ohio State Medical Society
Transactions of the Rhode Island Medical Society
Transactions of the Royal Society of Edinburgh
Transactions and Studies, College of Physicians of Philadelphia
Vermont History
Virginia Magazine of History and Biography
Water Cure Journal
Western Medical Reformer
Worcester Journal of Medicine

Books and Pamphlets

Abrahams, Harold J. *Extinct Medical Schools of Nineteenth Century Philadelphia*. Philadelphia: University of Pennsylvania Press, 1966.
Ackerknecht, Erwin H. *Medicine at the Paris Hospital, 1794–1848*. Baltimore: Johns Hopkins University Press, 1967.
———. *Rudolf Virchow: Doctor, Statesman, Anthropologist*. Madison: University of Wisconsin Press, 1953.
Agnew, D. Hayes. *The Principles and Practice of Surgery, Being a Treatise on Surgical Diseases and Injuries*. Philadelphia: J. B. Lippincott, 1878.
American Pharmaceutical Association. *The National Formulary of Unofficial Preparations*. Baltimore: American Pharmaceutical Association, 1896.
Annual Announcement of the Chicago Physio-Medical College. Chicago: William Johnston Printing, 1891.
Arber, Agnes. *Herbals, Their Origin and Evolution; A Chapter in the History of Botany, 1470–1670*. Darien: Hafner, 1970.
Ashhurst, John. *The Principles and Practice of Surgery*. Philadelphia: Lea Brothers, 1889.
Attfield, John. *Chemistry, General, Medical, and Pharmaceutical: Including the Chemistry of the U.S. Pharmacopoeia: A Manual on the General Principles of the Science, and Their Applications in Medicine and Pharmacy*. Philadelphia: Lea Brothers, 1889.
Baker, Samuel L. "Medical Licensing in America: An Early Liberal Reform." Ph.D. diss., Harvard University, 1977.
Bartlett, Elisha. *An Essay on the Philosophy of Medical Science*. Philadelphia: Lea and Blanchard, 1847.
———. *Inquiry Into the Degree of Certainty in Medicine; And Into the Nature and Extent of Its Power Over Disease*. Philadelphia: Lea and Blanchard, 1845.
Barton, Benjamin Smith. *Collections for an Essay Towards a Materia Medica of the United States*. Philadelphia: Way and Groff, 1798.

―――. *Elements of Botany; Or, Outlines of the Natural History of Vegetables.* Philadelphia: Printed for the Author, 1803.

Barton, William P. C. *The Vegetable Materia Medica of the United States; Or, Medica Botany.* 4 vols. Philadelphia: H. C. Carey and I. Lea, 1818–25.

Bastian, Henry C. *Beginnings of Life, Being Some Account of the Nature, Modes of Origin and Transformation of Lower Organisms.* 2 vols. New York: D. Appleton, 1872.

―――. *Evolution and the Origin of Life.* London: Macmillan, 1874.

Beach, Wooster. *The American Practice of Medicine; Being a Treatise on the Character, Causes, Symptoms, Morbid Appearances and Treatment of the Diseases of Men, Women and Children, of All Climates, on Vegetable or Botanical Principles.* 3 vols. New York: Betts and Anstice, 1833.

―――. *Beach's Family Physician and Home Guide: For the Treatment of the Diseases of Men, Women and Children on Reform Principles.* Cincinnati: Moore, Wilstach, Keys, 1860.

―――. *The Family Physician; Or, the Reformed System of Medicine: On Vegetable or Botanical Principles, Being a Compendium of the American Practice Designed for All Classes.* 5th ed. New York: Published for the Author, 1844.

Beale, Lionel Smith. *Disease Germs; Their Real Nature.* London: J. Churchill and Sons, 1870.

―――. *The Microscope in Medicine.* Philadelphia: Lindsay and Blakiston, 1878.

Beard, George Miller. *A Practical Treatise on Nervous Exhaustion (Neurasthenia): Its Symptoms, Nature, Sequences, Treatment.* New York: William Wood, 1880.

Bedford, Gunning S. *Clinical Lectures on the Diseases of Women and Children.* New York: W. Wood, 1856.

Benes, Peter. *Medicine and Healing; The Dublin Seminar for New England Folklife Annual Proceedings 1990.* Boston: Boston University Press, 1992.

Bennett, John Hughes. *Clinical Lectures on the Principles and Practice of Medicine.* 2d ed. New York: Samuel S. and William Wood, 1858.

―――. *The Pathology and Treatment of Pulmonary Tuberculosis; And on the Local Medication of Pharyngeal and Laryngeal Diseases Frequently Mistaken for, Or Associated With, Phthisis.* Philadelphia: Blanchard and Lea, 1854.

Berman, Alex. "The Impact of the Nineteenth Century Botanico-Medical Movement on American Pharmacy and Medicine." Ph.D. diss., Madison: University of Wisconsin, 1954.

―――. *A Striving for Scientific Respectability: Some American Botanics and the Nineteenth Century Plant Materia Medica.* Madison: American Institute of the History of Pharmacy, 1956.

Bigelow, Jacob. *American Medical Botany, Being a Collection of the Native Medicinal Plants of the United States.* 3 vols. Boston: Hilliard and Metcaff, 1817–20.

―――. *A Discourse on Self-Limited Diseases.* Boston: Hale, 1835.

Billroth, T. *The Medical Sciences in the German Universities: A Study in the History of Civilization.* New York: Macmillan, 1924.

Blackwell, Elizabeth. *Pioneer Work in Opening the Medical Profession to Women: Autobiographical Sketches*. London: Longman, Green, 1895.

Blanton, Wyndham B. *Medicine in Virginia in the Nineteenth Century*. Richmond: Garrett and Massie, 1933.

——. *Medicine in Virginia in the Seventeenth Century*. Richmond: William Byrd Press, 1930.

Blumenbach, Johann F. *The Institutes of Physiology*. Philadelphia: Benjamin Werner, 1817.

——. *Institutiones physiologicae*. Gottingen: J. C. Dieterich, 1798.

——. *Uber den Bildungstrieb*. Gottingen: J.C. Dieterich, 1789.

Bock, Hieronymus. *Kreuter Buch: darin underscheid Wurckung und Namen der Kreuter so in deutschen Landen washsen: auch der selben eigentlicher und wolgegrundter gebrauch inn der Artzney fleissig dargeben Leibs gesundheit*. Strassburg: Gedruckt bei W. Rihel, 1546.

Bodwitch, Henry I. *The Young Stethosopist; Or, the Student's Aid to Auscultation*. New York: Hafner, 1964.

Bonner, Thomas N. *Medicine in Chicago, a Chapter in the Social and Scientific Development of a City, 1850–1950*. Madison: American History Research Center, 1957.

Boorstin, Daniel J. *The Lost World of Thomas Jefferson*. Boston: Beacon Press, 1960.

Bowler, Peter J. *The Eclipse of Darwinism: Anti-Darwinian Evolution Theories in the Decades Around 1900*. Baltimore: Johns Hopkins University Press, 1983.

Boyle, Wade. *Herb Doctors: Pioneers in Nineteenth Century American Botanical Medicine and a History of the Eclectic Medical Institute of Cincinnati*. East Palestine, Ohio: Buckeye Naturopathic Press, 1988.

Brayton, James Harvey. "The Development of Medical Education in Indiana." Master's thesis, Indiana University, 1929.

Brieger, Gert H., ed. *Medical America in the Nineteenth Century*. Baltimore: Johns Hopkins University Press, 1972.

Brooks, Chandler, McC., and Paul E. Cranefield. *The Historical Development of Physiological Thought*. New York: Hafner, 1959.

Broussais, François J. V. *Principles on Physiological Medicine*. Philadelphia: H.C. Carey and I. Lea, 1832.

——. *A Treatise on Physiology*. Philadelphia: H.C. Carey and I. Lea, 1826.

Brown, John. *The Elements of Medicine; Or, A Translation of the Elementa Medicinae Brunonis With Large Notes, Illustrations and Comments*. London: J. Johnson, 1788.

Brown, Oliver P. *The Complete Herbalist; Or, the People Their Own Physicians by the Use of Nature's Remedies, and a New and Plain System of Hygienic Principles*. Jersey City, N.J.: The Author, 1872.

——. *The Complete Herbalist; Or, the People Their Own Physicians, by the Use of Nature's Remedies; Describing the Great Curative Properties Found in the*

Herbal Kingdom. A New and Plain System of Hygienic Principles. London: F. O. Hale, 1885.

Bryant, Joseph D. *Manual of Operative Surgery*. New York: D. Appleton, 1886.

Buchan, William. *Domestic Medicine, Or, A Treatise on the Prevention and Cure of Diseases, by Regimen and Simple Medicines*. 1769. 2d ed. Philadelphia: T. Dobson, 1797.

———. *Domestic Medicine; Or, the Family Physician; Being an Attempt to Render the Medical Art more Generally Useful, Chiefly Calculated to Recommend a Proper Attention to Regimen and Simple Medicines*. 1769. Philadelphia: Joseph Crukshank, 1774.

Bulloch, William. *The History of Bacteriology*. London: Oxford University Press, 1938.

Burkhalter, Lois Wood. *Gideon Lincecum, 1793–1874: A Biography*. Austin: University of Texas Press, 1965.

Burrow, James G. *AMA: Voice of American Medicine*. Baltimore: Johns Hopkins University Press, 1963.

Butterfield, Lyman H., ed. *Letters of Benjamin Rush*. 2 vols. Princeton, N.J.: Princeton University Press, 1951.

Byford, Henry T. *An American Textbook of Gynecology: Medical and Surgical*. Philadelphia: W. B. Saunders, 1893.

Bynum, W. F., and Roy Porter, eds. *Medical Fringe and Medical Orthodoxy, 1750–1850*. London: Croom Helm, 1987.

Cangi, Ellen Corwin. "Principles Before Practice: The Reform of Medical Education in Cincinnati Before and After the Flexner Report, 1870–1930." Ph.D. diss., University of Cincinnati, 1983.

Carpenter, J. Estlin, ed. *Nature and Man. Essays Scientific and Philosophical, by William B. Carpenter*. London: Kegan, Paul and Trench, 1888.

Carpenter, William B. *Elements of Physiology. Including Physiological Anatomy, For the Use of the Medical Student*. Philadelphia: Lea and Blanchard, 1846.

———. *Principles of Human Physiology*. London: J. Churchill, 1864.

———. *Principles of Physiology: General and Comparative*. 3d ed. London: Lea, 1851.

Carson, J. *History of the Medical Department of the University of Pennsylvania*. Philadelphia: Lindsay and Blakiston, 1869.

Carter, J. E. *The Botanic Physician and Family Medical Adviser and Dispensatory*. Madisonville, Tenn.: B. Parker, 1837.

Cash, Philip, Eric H. Christianson, and J. Worth Estes, eds. *Medicine in Colonial Massachusetts, 1620–1820*. Boston: Colonial Society of Massachusetts, 1980.

Cassedy, James H. *American Medical and Statistical Thinking, 1800–1860*. Cambridge: Harvard University Press, 1984.

———. *Medicine and American Growth, 1800–1860*. Madison: University of Wisconsin Press, 1986.

Castle, Thomas. *A Manual of Surgery, Founded Upon the Principles and Practice Lately Taught by Sir Astley Cooper and Joseph Henry Green*. London: E. Cox, 1839.

Cazeaux, Pierre. *A Theoretical and Practical Treatise on Midwifery*. Philadelphia: Lindsay and Blakiston, 1866.

Chailly-Honoré, Nicolas Charles. *Traité practique de l'art des accouchements*. New York: Harper and Brothers, 1844.

Channel, David F. *The Vital Machine: A Study of Technology and Organic Life*. New York: Oxford University Press, 1991.

Charcot, Jean-Martin. *Clinical Lectures on Certain Diseases of the Nervous System*. Detroit: Davis, 1888.

Chesney, A. M. *The Johns Hopkins Hospital and the Johns Hopkins University School of Medicine*. 3 vols. Baltimore: Johns Hopkins University Press, 1943, 1958, 1963.

Chomel, Auguste F. *Éléments de pathologie générale*. Paris: Fortin, Masson, 1841.

Churchill, Fleetwood. *On the Theory and Practice of Midwifery*. Philadelphia: Blanchard and Lea, 1851.

Clymer, Ruben Swineburne. *Nature's Healing Agents: The Medicines of Nature (or the Natura System)*. Quakertown, Pa.: Humanitarian Society, 1973.

———. *The Thomsonian System of Medicine: With Complete Rules for the Treatment of Disease: Also a Short Materia Medica*. Allentown, Pa.: Philosophical Publishing Company, 1906.

Coates, Reynell. *First Lines of Physiology*. Philadelphia: E. H. Butler, 1847.

Cobb, Daniel J. *The Medical Botanist and Treatment of Disease*. Castile, N.Y.: By the Author, 1846.

Colby, Benjamin. *A Guide to Health: Being an Exposition of the Principles of the Thomsonian System of Practice and Their Mode of Application in the Cure of Every Form of Disease; Embracing a Concise View of the Various Theories*. Nashua, N.H.: Charles T. Gill, 1844.

Colonial Society of Massachusetts. *Colonial Society in Massachusetts, 1620–1820*. Boston: Colonial Society of Massachusetts, 1980.

Comfort, John W. *The Practice of Medicine on Thomsonian Principles: Adapted as Well to the Use of Families as to That of the Practitioner: Containing a Biographical Sketch of Dr. Thomson: And a Materia Medica, Adapted to the Work*. 6th ed. Philadelphia: Lindsay and Blakiston, 1863.

———. *Thomsonian Instructor; Or, Practical Information on Thomsonian Medicines*. Philadelphia: Aaron Comfort, 1855.

———. *Thomsonian Practice of Medicine and Materia Medica*. Philadelphia: Aaron Comfort, 1842.

Cook, William H. *A Compend of the New Materia Medica Together With Additional Descriptions of Some Old Remedies*. Chicago: W. H. Cook, 1896.

———. *A Handbook of Family Medicine and Hygiene; Together With Descriptions of Remedies, Numerous Choice Formulas, Dietary for the Sick, Rules for Nursing, etc.* Cincinnati: George P. Houston, 1890.

————. *A Handbook of Practical Medicine: For the Use of Students, Practitioners and Families; Including a Formulary, Medical Ethics and Form of Will*. Cincinnati: W. H. Cook, 1859.

————. *Man: His Generative System and Marital Relations*. Cincinnati: W. H. Cook, 1890.

————. *The Physio-Medical Dispensatory: A Treatise on Therapeutics, Materia Medica, and Pharmacy, in Accordance With the Principles of Physiological Medication*. Cincinnati: By Author, 1869.

————. *A Treatise on the Principles and Practice of Physio-Medical Surgery; For the Use of Students and Practitioners*. Cincinnati: Moore, Wilstach, Keys, 1857.

————. *Woman's Book of Health: A Guide for the Wife, Mother, and Nurse*. Cincinnati: William W. Cook, 1884.

———— *Woman's Handbook of Health*. Cincinnati: The Author, 1866.

Cook, William Wesley. *Practical Lessons in Hypnotism, Containing Complete Instructions in the Development and Practice of Hypnotic Power, Including Much Valuable Information in Regard to Mental Healing, Mind Reading and Other Kindred Subjects*. Chicago: Thompson and Thomas, 1901.

Cornil, Victor. *Syphilis*. Philadelphia: Henry C. Lea's Son, 1882.

Coulter, Harris L. *Divided Legacy: A History of Schism in Medical Thought. Vol. 3. Science and Ethics in Medicine: 1800–1914*. Washington, D.C.: Wehawken, 1973.

Cullen, William. *Institutions of Medicine, Part 1: Physiology*. 3d ed. Edinburgh: C. Elliot, 1785.

Culpeper, Nicholas. *Complete Herbal, and English Physician: Wherein Several Hundred Herbs, With a Display of Their Medicinal and Occult Properties are Physically Applied to the Cure of All Disorders Incident to Mankind*. Manchester: J. Gleave, 1826.

————. *The English Physician Enlarged, Containing 300 Medicines, Made of American Herbs. Being an Astrologo-Physical Discourse of the Vulger Herbs of This Nation, Containing a Complete Method of Physic*. Leeds: Printed for John Binns, 1799.

————. *Pharmacopoeia Londinensis, or the London Dispensatory*. London, 1649.

Curtis, Alva. *Allopathy and Physio-Medication Contrasted*. Cincinnati: By the Author, 1867.

————. *Discussions Between Several Members of the Regular Medical Faculty and the Thomsonian Botanic Physicians*. Columbus, Ohio: Alva Curtis, 1835.

————. *A Fair Examination and Criticism of All the Medical Systems in Vogue*. 2d ed. Cincinnati: Printed for the Proprietor, 1865.

————. *Lectures on Midwifery and the Forms of Disease Peculiar to Women and Children: Delivered to the Members of the Botanico-Medical College of Ohio*. Columbus, Ohio: Printed for the Author, 1841.

————. *The Provocation and the Reply; Or, Allopathy Versus Physio-Medicalism in a Review of Prof. M.B. Wright's Remarks at the Dedication of the Cincinnati*

New Hospital, January 8th, 1869. Cincinnati: Published for the Proprietor, 1870.

———. *Synopsis of a Course of Lectures on Medical Science, Delivered to the Students of the Botanico-Medical College of Ohio*. Cincinnati: Edwin Shepard, 1846.

———. *A Synopsis of Lectures on Medical Science; Embracing the Principles of Medicine, or Physiology, Pathology, and Therapeutics, as Discovered in Nature; and the Practice According to Those Principles, as Applied by Art*. 7th ed. New York: A. J. Graham, 1877.

Dadd, G. H. *American Cattle Doctor*. New York: C. M. Saxton, 1855.

Dale, W. *The Principles and Practice of the Botanic System of Medicine*. Glasgow: Murray, 1855.

Dalton, John C. *A Treatise on Human Physiology: Designed for the Use of Students and Practitioners of Medicine*. Philadelphia: Henry C. Lea, 1871.

Darwin, Charles. *On the Origin of Species by Means of Natural Selection, Or, the Preservation of Favoured Races in the Struggle for Life*. London: J. Murray, 1859.

Davis, David J., ed. *History of Medical Practice in Illinois. Volume 2: 1850–1900*. Chicago: Illinois State Medical Society, 1955.

Davis, Henry G. *Conservative Surgery, as Exhibited in Remedying Some of the Mechanical Causes that Operate Injuriously Both in Health and Disease*. New York: D. Appleton, 1867.

Davis, Nathan S. *Clinical Lectures on Various Important Diseases; Being a Collection of the Clinical Lectures Delivered in the Medical Wards of Mercy Hospital, Chicago*. Chicago: J. J. Spalding, 1873.

———. *Contributions to the History of Medical Education and Medical Institutions in the United States of America, 1776–1876*. Washington, D.C.: Government Printing Office, 1877.

Day, L. Meeker. *The Botanic Family Physician; Or, the Secret of Curing All Diseases on Improved Hygeian Principles, Fully Disclosed, Together With a Valuable Digest on Midwifery*. New York: n.p., 1833.

Day, William H. *Essays on Diseases of Children*. London: J. and A. Churchill, 1873.

de Bordeu, Theophile. *Oeuvres completes*. Paris: Caille et Ravier, 1767.

Dennert, E. *At the Deathbed of Darwinism*. Burlington, Iowa: German Literary Board, 1904.

Derbyshire, Robert C. *Medical Licensure and Discipline in the United States*. Baltimore: Johns Hopkins University Press, 1969.

Dercum, Francis Xavier. *Rest, Mental Therapeutics, and Suggestion*. Philadelphia: P. Blakiston's Son, 1903.

de Sauvages, François Boissier. *Physiologiae elementa*. Amsterdam: J. Tilan, 1755.

Drake, Daniel. *Discourse on the History, Character, and Prospects of the West*. Gainesville, Fla.: Scholars' Facsimiles and Reprints, 1955.

Draper, John William. *Human Physiology, Statical and Dynamical; Or, the Conditions and Course of the Life of Man*. New York: Harper and Brothers, 1856.

Dressler, Florence. *Feminology; A Guide for Womankind, Giving in Detail Instructions as to Motherhood, Maidenhood, and the Nursery*. Chicago: C. L. Dressler, 1902.

Driesch, Hans. *Gifford Lectures Delivered Before the University of Aberdeen in the Years 1907 and 1908*. 2 vols. London: Adam and Charles Black, 1908.

———. *The History and Theory of Vitalism*. London: Macmillan, 1914.

———. *The Problem of Individuality: A Course of Four Lectures Delivered Before the University of London in October 1913*. London: Macmillan, 1914.

Druitt, Robert. *The Principles and Practice of Modern Surgery*. Philadelphia: Blanchard and Lea, 1856.

Duffy, John. *The Healers: The Rise of the Medical Establishment*. New York: McGraw-Hill, 1976.

Duhring, Louis A. *A Practical Treatise on Diseases of the Skin*. Philadelphia: J. B. Lippincott, 1877.

Dunbar, Newall. *The "Elixir of Life"—Dr. Brown-Sequard's Own Account of His Famous Alleged Remedy for Debility and Old Age, Dr. Variot's Experiments, and Contemporaneous Comments of the Profession and the Press*. Boston: J. G. Cupples, 1889.

Dunglison, Robley. *History of Medicine, From the Earliest Ages to the Commencement of the Nineteenth Century*. Philadelphia: Lindsay and Blakistan, 1872.

Dunham, William R. *Theory of Medical Science: The Doctrine of an Inherent Power in Medicine a Fallacy: The Ultimate Special Properties of Vitality and the Laws of Vital Force Constitute the Fundamental Basis of Medical Philosophy and Science*. Boston: James Campbell, 1876.

Dunsch, Lothar. *Ein Fundament zum Gebaude der Wissenschaften: Einhundret Jahre Ostwald's Klassiker der Exakten Wissenschaften*. Leipzig: Geest and Portig, 1889.

Dwyer, M. Virginia, ed. *American Medical Directory*. 20th ed. Chicago: American Medical Association, 1958.

Earle, A. Scott, ed. *Surgery in America from the Colonial Era to the Twentieth Century*. 2d ed. New York: Praeger, 1983.

Eaton, Amos. *Manual of Botany, for North America: Containing Generic and Specific Descriptions of the Indigenous Plants and Common Cultivated Exotics, Growing North of the Gulf of Mexico*. 5th ed. Albany: Websters and Skinners, 1829.

Edwards, J. Jep. *A Compend of Physio-Medical Treatment*. Columbus, Ind.: Edwards Brothers, 1895.

Edwards, Joseph F. *How We Ought to Live*. Philadelphia: H. C. Watts, 1882.

Eisley, Loren. *Darwin's Century: Evolution and the Men Who Discovered It*. New York: Doubleday, 1958.

Emmett, Thomas A. *The Principles and Practice of Gynaecology*. Philadelphia: H. C. Lea, 1879.

Erichsen, John Eric. *The Science and Art of Surgery: A Treatise on Surgical Injuries, Diseases, and Operations*. 2 vols. Philadelphia: Henry C. Lea's Son, 1884–85.

Estes, J. Worth. *Dictionary of Protopharmacology: Therapeutic Practices, 1700–1850*. Canton, Mass.: Science History Publications, 1990.

Estes, J. Worth, and David M. Goodman. *The Changing Humors of Portsmouth: The Medical Biography of an American Town, 1623–1983*. Boston: Francis A. Countway Library of Medicine, 1986.

Faculty of the Reform Medical College of Georgia. *The Reform-Medical Practice: With a History of Medicine, From the Earliest Period to the Present Time, and a Synopsis of Principles on Which the New Practice is Founded*. Macon, Ga.: M. S. Thomson, 1857.

Farley, John. *The Spontaneous Generation Controversy: From Descartes to Oparin*. Baltimore: Johns Hopkins University Press, 1977.

Fellows, Otis E., and Stephen F. Milliken. *Buffon*. New York: Twayne, 1972.

Felter, Harvey Wickes. *History of the Eclectic Medical Institute, Cincinnati, Ohio, 1845–1902*. Cincinnati: Alumnal Association, 1902.

Fiske, John. *Outlines of Cosmic Philosophy*. 4 vols. Boston: Houghton Mifflin, 1903.

Flexner, Abraham. *Medical Education in the United States and Canada; A Report to the Carnegie Foundation on the Advancement of Teaching*. New York: Carnegie Foundation, 1910.

Flexner, Simon. *The Evolution and Organization of the University Clinic*. Oxford: Clarendon Press, 1939.

Flint, Austin. *Physical Exploration and Diagnoses of Diseases Affecting the Respiratory Organs*. Philadelphia: Blanchard and Lea, 1856.

————. *A Practical Treatise on the Diagnosis, Pathology, and Treatment of Diseases of the Heart*. Philadelphia: Blanchard and Lea, 1859.

————. *A Text-Book of Human Physiology; Designed for the Use of Practitioners and Students of Medicine*. New York: D. Appleton, 1876.

————. *A Treatise on the Principles and Practice of Medicine; Designed for the Use of Practitioners and Students of Medicine*. Philadelphia: H. C. Lea, 1866.

Fonerden, William H. *The Institutes of Thomsonianism*. Philadelphia: n.p., 1837.

Foster, Sir Michael. *A Textbook of Physiology*. London: Macmillan, 1878.

Foster, William D. *A History of Medical Bacteriology and Immunology*. London: William Heinemann Medical, 1970.

Fothergill, John Milner. *The Will Power: Its Range in Action*. Cleveland, Ohio: P. W. Garfield, 1889.

Fownes, George. *Elementary Chemistry, Theoretical and Practical*. Philadelphia: Lea and Blanchard, 1847.

Fox, Henry. *Photographic Atlas of the Diseases of the Skin; With Descriptive Text and a Treatise on Cutaneous Therapeutics*. Philadelphia: J. B. Lippincott, 1902.

Fox, William, and Joseph Nadin. *The Working Man's Family Botanic Guide*. Sheffield: Dawson, 1852.

Freyhofer, Horst H. *The Vitalism of Hans Driesch; The Success and Decline of a Scientific Theory*. Frankfurt: Peter Lang, 1982.

Friend, J. D., and H. M. Sweet, eds. *The American Journal of Medical Reform, for the People and the Profession*. New York: H. Winchester, 1857.

Fuchs, Leonard. *De historia stirpium commentarii insignes, maximis impensis et vigiliis elaborati, adjectis erundem vivis plusquam quingentis imaginibus*. Basileae: In Officina Isingriniana, 1542.

Fuller, Robert C. *Alternative Medicine and American Religious Life*. New York: Oxford University Press, 1989.

Gallup, Joseph A. *Outlines of the Institutes of Medicine; Founded on the Philosophy of Human Economy, in Health, and in Disease*. Boston: Otis, Broaders, 1839.

Garrison, Fielding H. *Introduction to the History of Medicine*. 4th ed. Philadelphia: W. B. Saunders, 1929.

Gerhard, William W. *On the Diagnoses of Diseases of the Chest; Based Upon the Comparison of Their Physical and General Signs*. Philadelphia: Key and Biddle, 1836.

Gevitz, Norman, ed. *Other Healers; Unorthodox Medicine in America*. Baltimore: Johns Hopkins University Press, 1988.

Gillespie, Neal. *Charles Darwin and the Problem of Creation*. Chicago: University of Chicago Press, 1979.

Goler, Robert I., and Pascal James Imperato, eds. *Early American Medicine: A Symposium*. New York: Fraunces Tavern Museum, 1987.

Goodfield, G. F. *The Growth of Scientific Physiology; Physiological Method and the Mechanist-Vitalist Controversy*. London: Hutchinson, 1960.

Graves, Robert. *Clinical Lectures*. New York: J. and H. G. Langley, 1842.

Gray, Asa. *First Lessons in Botany and Vegetable Physiology*. New York: Ivisan, 1866.

———. *Manual of Botany of the Northern United States, Including the District East of the Mississippi and North of North Carolina and Tennessee, Arranged According to the Natural System*. New York: Ivisan, 1868.

Gray, Henry. *Anatomy, Descriptive and Surgical*. Philadelphia: Henry C. Lea's Son, 1883.

Gray, John F. *Early Annals of Homoeopathy in New York*. New York: W. S. Door, 1865.

Gregory, Frederick. *Scientific Materialism in Nineteenth Century Germany*. Dordrecht: Reidel, 1977.

Gross, Samuel D. *Elements of Pathological Anatomy*. Philadelphia: Blanchard and Lea, 1857.

———. *A System of Surgery; Pathological, Diagnostic, Therapeutique, and Operative*. Philadelphia: Blanchard and Lea, 1859.

Hahnemann, Samuel. *The Chronic Diseases: Their Specific Nature and Their Homeopathic Treatment*. New York: William Raddle, 1845.

———. *Materia Medica Pura*. Liverpool: Hahnemann Publishing Society, 1880–81.

————. *Organon of Homoeopathic Medicine*. New York: Radde, 1843.

Hall, Marshall. *Observations on Blood-Letting Founded Upon Researches on the Morbid and Curative Effects of Loss of Blood*. London: Sherwood, 1836.

————. *Principles of the Theory and Practice of Medicine*. Boston: C.C. Little and J. Brown, 1839.

Hall, Thomas S. *Ideas of Life and Matter; Studies in the History of General Physiology, 600 B.C.–1900 A.D.* 2 vols. Chicago: University of Chicago Press, 1969.

Haller, Albrecht von. *A Dissertation on the Sensible and Irritable Parts of Animals*. Baltimore: Johns Hopkins University Press, 1936.

————. *First Lines of Physiology*. Edinburgh: Bell and Bradfute, 1801.

Haller, John S., Jr. *American Medicine in Transition, 1840–1910*. Urbana: University of Illinois Press, 1981.

————. *Medical Protestants: The Eclectics in American Medicine, 1825–1939*. Carbondale: Southern Illinois University Press, 1994.

Hamilton, Frank Hastings. *The Principles and Practice of Surgery*. New York: William Wood, 1872.

Hammond, William A. *A Treatise on the Diseases of the Nervous System*. New York: D. Appleton, 1891.

————. *A Treatise on Insanity in Its Medical Relations*. 1883. New York: Arno Press, 1973.

Hard, M. K. *Woman's Medical Guide; Being a Complete Review of the Peculiarities of the Female Constitution, and the Derangements to Which It Is Subject, With a Description of Simple Yet Certain Means for Their Cure*. Mt. Vernon, Ohio: W.W. Cochran, 1848.

Harrison, Robert. *The Surgical Anatomy of the Arteries of the Human Body*. New York: J. and H. G. Langley, 1840.

Hartshorne, Henry. *Essentials of the Principles and Practice of Medicine*. Philadelphia: H. C. Lea, 1867.

Harvey, A. McGehee. *Adventures in Medical Research: A Century of Discovery at Johns Hopkins*. Baltimore: Johns Hopkins University Press, 1976.

————. *Science at the Bedside: Clinical Research in American Medicine, 1905–1945*. Baltimore: Johns Hopkins University Press, 1981.

Hein, Wolfgang-Gagen, ed. *Botanical Drugs of the Americas in the Old and New Worlds*. Stuttgart: Wissenschaftliche Verlagsgesellschaft MBH, 1984.

Heitzmann, Carl. *The Cell-Doctrine in the Light of Recent Investigations*. New York: D. Appleton, 1877.

Henry, Samuel. *A New and Complete Family Herbal*. New York: Samuel Henry, 1814.

Higby, Gregory J., ed. *One Hundred Years of the National Formulary: A Symposium*. Madison, Wis.: American Institute of the History of Pharmacy, 1989.

Hill, James. *Cases in Surgery, Particularly of Cancers, and Disorders of the Head from External Violence, With Observations*. Edinburgh: J. Balfour, 1772.

Hoener, Frederick G. *The New Physiologic Medication*. 2d ed. Baltimore: F. G. Hoener, 1900.

Hooker, Worthington. *Dissertation on the Respect Due to the Medical Profession, and the Reasons Why It is Not Awarded by the Community*. Norwich: J. G. Cooley, 1844.

————. *Physician and Patient; Or, a Practical View of the Mutual Duties, Relations, and Interests of the Medical Profession and the Community*. New York: Baker and Scribner, 1849.

Horner, William E. *Special Anatomy and Histology*. Philadelphia: Blanchard, 1851.

House, Eleazer G. *The Botanic Family Friend: Being a Complete Guide to the New System of Thomsonian Medical Practice*. Boston: Printed for the Author, 1844.

Howard, Horton. *An Improved System of Botanic Medicine Founded Upon Correct Physiological Principles; Comprising a Complete Treatise on the Practice of Medicine*. Cincinnati: Kost, Bigger and Hart, 1832.

————. *An Improved System of Botanic Medicine: Founded Upon Correct; Together With an Illustration of the New Theory of Medicine*. 3d ed., 3 vols. Columbus, Ohio: Published by the Proprietors, 1836.

Howe, Joseph W. *Emergencies, and How to Treat Them. The Etiology, Pathology, and Treatment of the Accidents, Diseases, and Cases of Poisoning Which Demand Prompt Action*. New York: D. Appleton, 1871.

Hudson, Thomson Jay. *The Law of Psychic Phenomena*. Chicago: A. C. McClurg, 1893.

Huxley, Thomas Henry. *Science and Education*. New York: Appleton, 1894.

Hyman, Max R. *Journal Handbook of Indianapolis*. Indianapolis: Indianapolis Journal Newspaper Company, 1902.

Illinois State Board of Health. *Report on Medical Education and the Regulation of the Practice of Medicine in the United States and Canada*. Springfield, Ill.: State Board of Health, 1883.

Jahr, Gottlieb Heinrich. *Hull's Jahr; A New Manual of Homeopathic Practice*. New York: W. Radde, 1862.

Juettner, Otto. *Daniel Drake and His Followers: Historical and Biographical Sketches*. Cincinnati: Harvey Publishing Company, 1909.

Kaufman, Martin. "American Medical Education." In *The Education of American Physicians*, ed. Ronald Numbers. Berkeley: University of California Press, 1980.

————. *American Medical Education: The Formative Years, 1765–1910*. Westport, Conn.: Greenwood Press, 1976.

Kaufman, Martin, Stewart Gailishoff, and Todd L. Savitt, eds., *Dictionary of American Medical Biography*. 2 vols. Westport, Conn.: Greenwood Press, 1984.

Keith, Melville C. *Childbirth and the Child. A Treatise for Parents and Nurses on the Care of the Mother and Child, During Gestation, Pregnancy and Parturition.* Minneapolis, Minn.: Alfred Roper, 1888.

————. *Diphtheria: Its History, Symptoms, Causes, Prevention and Cure. Scarlet Fever and Its Successful Treatment.* Lincoln, Neb.: S. L. Moser, 1879.

————. *Forms of Fever, Especially Typhoid; With Radical Treatment and Formulas for the Speedy Curing of All Cases of Fever of Every Kind.* Bellville, Ohio: Keith, 1898.

————. *Keith's Domestic Practice and Botanic Hand Book.* Bellville, Ohio: Published by the Author, 1901.

————. *The Marriage Law: A Medical and Philosophical Treatise on the Marital Habits of the Human Race and the Rights of Sexual Compact Between the Sexes: The Law and the Testimony.* Bellville, Ohio: Keith, 1913.

Kett, F. Joseph. *The Formation of the American Medical Profession: The Role of Institutions, 1750–1860.* New Haven: Yale University Press, 1968.

King, John. *The American Eclectic Dispensatory.* 1859. 8th ed. Cincinnati: Moore, Wilstach, Keys, 1870.

Konold, Donald E. *A History of American Medical Ethics, 1847–1912.* Madison: University of Wisconsin Press, 1962.

Kost, John. *Domestic Medicine; A Treatise on the Practice of Medicine Adapted to the Reformed System, Comprising a Materia Medica.* Cincinnati: Burnard, 1851.

————. *Elements of the Materia Medica and Therapeutics: Adapted to the New Physiological System of Practice.* Cincinnati: Kost and Pool, 1849.

————. *The Practice of Medicine According to the Plan Most Approved by the Reformed or Botanic Colleges of the United States, Embracing a Treatise on Materia Medica and Pharmacy, Designed Principally for Families.* Mt. Vernon, Ohio: n.p., 1847.

Lamarck, Jean Baptiste. *Histoire naturelle des animaux sans vertebres.* Paris: Verdiere, 1815.

————. *Zoological Philosophy.* New York: Hafner, 1963.

La Mettrie, Julien Offrey de. *L'homme machine.* Princeton: Princeton University Press, 1960.

Leavitt, Judith W., and Ronald L. Numbers, eds. *Sickness and Health in America: Readings in the History of Medicine and Public Health.* Madison: University of Wisconsin Press, 1985.

Lechevalier, H. A., and M. Solotorovsky. *Three Centuries of Microbiology.* New York: McGraw-Hill, 1965.

Leighton, Ann. *Early American Gardens: For Meate or Medicine.* Worcester: American Antiquarian Society, 1970.

Lenoir, Timothy. *The Strategy of Life: Teleology and Mechanics in Nineteenth Century German Biology.* Dordrecht: D. Reidel, 1982.

Lewin, George R. *The Treatment of Syphilis With Subcutaneous Sublimate Injections.* Philadelphia: Lindsay and Blakiston, 1872.

Lincecum, Gideon. *Lincecum Papers*. Located at Barker Texas History Center, University of Texas at Austin.

Lincecum, Jerry Bryan, and Edward Hake Phillips, eds. *Adventures of a Frontier Naturalist; The Life and Times of Dr. Gideon Lincecum*. College Station: Texas A&M University Press, 1994.

Liston, Robert. *Practical Surgery*. Philadelphia: A. Waldie, 1838.

Lloyd, John Uri. *The Eclectic Alkaloids, Resins, Resinoids, Oleo-Resins and Concentrated Principle*. Cincinnati: J. U. and C. G. Lloyd, 1910.

―――. *History of the Vegetable Drugs of the Pharmacopoeia of the United States*. Cincinnati: J. U. and C. G. Lloyd, 1911.

―――. *Origin and History of All the Pharmacopeial Vegetable Drugs, Chemicals and Preparations*. Cincinnati: Caxton Press, 1921.

Loomis, Alfred L. *A Textbook of Practical Medicine*. New York: W. Wood, 1884.

Lopate, Carol. *Women in Medicine*. Baltimore: Johns Hopkins University Press, 1968.

Ludmerer, Kenneth M. *Learning to Heal: The Development of American Medical Education*. New York: Basic Books, 1985.

Lusk, William Thompson. *The Science and Art of Midwifery*. New York: D. Appleton, 1892.

Lyle, T. J. *Physio-Medical Therapeutics, Materia Medica, and Pharmacy*. Salem, Ohio: J. M. Lyle and Brothers, 1897.

Macfie, Ronald C. *Heredity, Evolution, and Vitalism: Some of the Discoveries of Modern Research Into These Matters—Their Trends and Significance*. Bristol: John Wright and Sons, 1912.

Marshall, Humphrey. *Arbustrum americanum: the American grove, or, An alphabetical catalogue of forest trees and shrubs, natives of the American United States, arranged according to the Linnaean system*. Philadelphia: Printed by J. Crukshank, 1785.

Massie, J. M. *The Advanced School of Medicine*. Dallas, Texas: n.p., 1892.

Mather, Cotton. *The Angel of Bethesda, Visiting the Invalids of a Miserable World*. New London, Conn.: Printed and Sold by Timothy Green, 1722.

Mattson, Morris. *The American Vegetable Practice, Or, A New and Improved Guide to Health, Designed for the Use of Families*. 2 vols. Boston: Daniel L. Hale, 1841.

Maudsley, Henry. *The Pathology of Mind*. London: Macmillan, 1879.

Maygrier, Jacques Pierre. *Midwifery Illustrated*. New York: Harper and Brothers, 1834.

Meigs, Charles D. *Obstetrics, the Science and the Art*. Philadelphia: Blanchard and Lea, 1849.

Metzger, Helene. *Newton, Stahl, Boerhaave et la doctrine chimique*. Paris: Alcan, 1930.

Meyer, Édouard. *A Practical Treatise on Diseases of the Eye*. Philadelphia: P. Blakiston, Son, 1887.

Miller, Amy B. *Shaker Herbs—a History and a Compendium*. New York: C. N. Potter, 1976.

Moll, Albert. *Hypnotism*. New York: Scribner and Welford, 1890.

Morantz-Sanchez, Regina M. *Sympathy and Science: Women Physicians in American Medicine*. New York: Oxford University Press, 1985.

Morton, Samuel, and William Cadge. *The Surgical Anatomy of the Principal Regions of the Human Body*. London: Taylor, Walton and Marberly, 1850.

Müller, Johannes. *Elements of Physiology*. New York: Leavitt, 1852.

Murphy, Lamar R. *Enter the Physician: The Transformation of Domestic Medicine, 1760–1860*. Tuscaloosa: University of Alabama Press, 1991.

Myers, Burton D. *The History of Medical Education in Indiana*. Bloomington: University of Indiana Press, 1956.

Neumann, Isidor. *Hand-Book of Skin Diseases*. New York: D. Appleton, 1872.

Nineteenth Annual Announcement of the Physio-Medical College of Indiana. Indianapolis: Baker-Randolph Company, 1891.

Nissenbaum, Stephen. *Sex, Diet, and Debility in Jacksonian America: Sylvester Graham and Health Reform*. Westport, Conn.: Greenwood Press, 1980.

Nordenskiold, Erik. *The History of Biology*. New York: Tudor, 1946.

Norwood, William F. *Medical Education in the United States Before the Civil War*. Philadelphia: University of Pennsylvania Press, 1944.

Numbers, Ronald, ed. *The Education of American Physicians*. Berkeley: University of California Press, 1980.

Oliver, Daniel. *First Lines of Physiology; Designed for the Use of Students of Medicine*. Philadelphia: Hooker and Agnew, 1841.

Parkes, Edmund A. *Public Health*. London: J. and A. Churchill, 1876.

Parrish, Edward. *An Introduction to Practical Pharmacy*. Philadelphia: Blanchard and Lea, 1856.

Parvin, Theophilus. *The Science and Art of Obstetrics*. Philadelphia: Lea Brothers, 1886.

Payne, Joseph F. *A Manual of General Pathology Designed as an Introduction to the Practice of Medicine*. Philadelphia: Lea Brothers, 1888.

Pepper, William. *A System of Practical Medicine*. 5 vols. Philadelphia: Lea Brothers, 1885–86.

———. *A Textbook of the Theory and Practice of Medicine*. 2 vols. Philadelphia: W. B. Saunders, 1894–95.

Phillips, Clifton J. *Indiana in Transition; The Emergence of an Industrial Commonwealth, 1880–1920*. Indianapolis: Indiana Historical Bureau and Indiana Historical Society, 1968.

Pickard, Madge E., and R. Carlyle Buley. *The Midwest Pioneer; His Ills, Cures, and Doctors*. New York: Henry Schuman, 1946.

Playfair, William Smoult. *A Treatise on the Science and Practice of Midwifery*. 2 vols. London: Smith, Elder, 1886.

Polk's Medical Register and Directory of North America. Detroit: R. L. Polk, 1886–1906.

Poynter, F. N. L. *Medicine and Science in the 1860s: Proceedings of the 6th British Congress on the History of Medicine.* London: Welcome Institute for the History of Medicine, 1968.

Quain, Jones. *Elements of Anatomy.* London: Bradbury, Agnew, 1828.

Radl, Emmanuel. *The History of Biological Theories.* Oxford: Oxford University Press, 1930.

Rafinesque, Constantine S. *Medical Flora: Or, Manual of the Medical Botany of the United States of North America.* 2 vols. Philadelphia: Atkinson and Alexander, 1828–30.

Ranney, Ambrose L. *A Practical Treatise on Surgical Diagnosis. Designed as a Manual for Practitioners and Students.* New York: W. Wood, 1881.

Ranvier, Louis Antoine, and André-Victor Cornil. *A Manual of Pathology and Histology.* Philadelphia: n.p., 1880.

Rather, L. J. *Disease, Life, and Man, Selected Essays by Rudolph Virchow.* Stanford: Stanford University Press, 1958.

Ray, Isaac. *A Treatise on the Medical Jurisprudence of Insanity.* New York: Arno Press, 1976 [1871].

Reed, Louis S. *The Healing Cults; A Study of Sectarian Medical Practice: Its Extent, Causes, and Control.* Chicago: University of Chicago Press, 1932.

Ringer, Sidney. *A Handbook of Therapeutics.* New York: W. Wood, 1878.

Risse, Guenter B., Ronald L. Numbers, and Judith W. Leavitt, eds. *Medicine Without Doctors; Home Health Care in American History.* New York: Science History Publications, 1977.

Ritterbush, Philip C. *Overtures to Biology: The Speculations of Eighteenth Century Naturalists.* New Haven: Yale University Press, 1964.

Roberts, Frederick T. *A Handbook of the Theory and Practice of Medicine.* Philadelphia: Lindsay and Blakistan, 1874.

Robinson, Samuel. *A Course of Fifteen Lectures, on Medical Botany, Denominated Thomson's New Theory of Medical Practice; in Which the Various Theories That Have Preceded It Are Reviewed and Compared; Delivered in Cincinnati, Ohio.* Columbus: Horton Howard, 1829.

Rockwell, Alphonso David. *Lectures on Electricity in Its Relations to Medicine and Surgery.* New York: William Wood, 1879.

Roe, Shirley A. *Matter, Life, and Generation: Eighteenth Century Embryology and the Haller-Wolff Debate.* Cambridge: Cambridge University Press, 1981.

———, ed. *The Natural Philosophy of Albrecht von Haller.* New York: Arno Press, 1981.

Rokitansky, Karl. *A Manual of Pathological Anatomy.* London: Sydenham Society, 1849–54.

Roosa, D. B. St. John. *A Practical Treatise on the Diseases of the Ear: Including the Anatomy of the Organ.* New York: William Wood, 1873.

Roscoe, Henry E. *Lessons in Elementary Chemistry, Inorganic and Organic*. New York: W. Wood, 1868.

Rosenfield, Leonora D. C. *From Beast-Machine to Man-Machine: Animal Soul in French Letters from Descartes to La Mettrie.* New York: Oxford University Press, 1941.

Rothstein, William G. *American Physicians in the Nineteenth Century: From Sects to Science*. Baltimore: Johns Hopkins University Press, 1972.

Rush, Benjamin. *Medical Injuries and Observations*. 2d ed. 4 vols. Philadelphia: J. Conrad, 1789.

Scarborough, John, ed. *Folklore and Folk Medicines*. Madison, Wis.: American Institute of the History of Medicine, 1987.

Schafer, Edward Albert. *Quain's Elements of Anatomy*. London: Longmans, Green, 1898.

Schoepf, Johann David. *Materia medica americana potissimum regni vegetabilis*. Erlangae: Palmii, 1787.

Schofield, Robert E. *Mechanism and Materialism: British Natural Philosophy in an Age of Reason*. Princeton, N.J.: Princeton University Press, 1970.

Scudder, John M. *Specific Diagnosis: A Study of Disease with Special Reference to the Administration of Remedies*. Cincinnati: Wilstach, Baldwin, 1874.

———. *Specific Medication and Specific Medicines*. Cincinnati: Wilstach, Baldwin, 1870.

Shafer, Henry B. *The American Medical Profession: 1783–1850*. New York: Columbia University Press, 1936.

Shryock, Richard H. *The Development of Modern Medicine; An Interpretation of the Social and Scientific Factors Involved*. Philadelphia: University of Pennsylvania Press, 1936.

———. *Medical Licensing in America, 1650–1965*. Baltimore: Johns Hopkins University Press, 1967.

Sims, James Marion. *Clinical Notes on Uterine Surgery*. New York: W. Wood, 1869.

Skelton, John. *The Epitome of the Botanic Practice of Medicine*. Leeds: Samuel Moxon, 1855.

———. *Family Medical Adviser*. Leeds: Moxon and Walker, 1852.

———. *A Plea for the Botanic Practice of Medicine*. London: Watson, 1853.

Skene, Alexander J. C. *Treatise on the Diseases of Women: For the Use of Students and Practitioners*. New York: D. Appleton, 1888.

Skoda, Joseph. *Abhandlung uber Perkussion und Auskultation. Sechste, theilweise umgerarbeitete und vermehrte Auflang*. Wien: L. W. Seidel and Sohn, 1864.

Slack, George. *Treatise on the Pathology of Disease*. 5th ed. London: J. Burns, 1891.

Sloan, Philip R., and J. Lyon, eds. *From Natural History to the History of Nature: Readings from Buffon and His Critics*. Notre Dame, Ind.: University of Notre Dame Press, 1981.

Smith, Elias. *The American Physician and Family Assistant*. Boston: E. Bellamy, 1826.

———. *The Medical Pocket-Book. Family Physician and Sick Man's Guide to Health*. Boston: Henry Bowen, 1822.

Smith, Elisha. *The Botanic Physician; Being a Compendium of the Practice of Physic, Upon Botanical Principles*. New York: Murphy and Bingham, 1830.

Smith, Eustace. *A Practical Treatise on Disease in Children*. Philadelphia: P. Blakiston, Son, 1887.

Smith, Norman Kemp. *New Studies in the Philosophy of Descartes*. London: Macmillan, 1952.

Sonnedecker, Glenn. *Kremers and Urdang's History of Pharmacy*. 3d ed. Philadelphia: J. B. Lippincott, 1963.

Sperry, I. J. *Family Medical Adviser; Containing a Complete History of Disease, With the Method and Mode of Cure*. Hartford, Conn.: J. G. Wells, 1847.

Stahl, George E. *Theoria medica vera*. Halle: Liferis Orphanotrophei, 1709.

Starr, Louis. *Diseases of the Digestive Organs in Infancy and Childhood*. Philadelphia: P. Blakiston, Son, 1886.

Starr, Paul E. *The Social Transformation of American Medicine: The Rise of a Sovereign Profession and the Making of a Vast Industry*. New York: Basic Books, 1982.

Stevens, John. *Medical Reform; Or Physiology and Botanic Practice for the People*. London: Whittaker, 1848.

Stillé, Alfred. *The National Dispensatory: Containing the Natural History, Chemistry, Pharmacy, Actions, and Uses of Medicines; Including Those Recognized in the Pharmacopoeias of the United States, Great Britain, and Germany, With Numerous References to the French Codex*. Philadelphia: Henry C. Lea's Son, 1886.

Stowell, Charles H. *The Student's Manual of Histology for the Use of Students, Practitioners and Microscopists*. Ann Arbor: C. H. Stowell, 1884.

Swanzy, Henry R. *A Handbook of the Diseases of the Eye and Their Treatment*. London: H. K. Lewis, 1884.

Taylor, Alfred Swaine. *On Poisons in Relation to Medical Jurisprudence and Medicine*. Philadelphia: Blanchard and Lea, 1859.

———. *Taylor's Principles and Practice of Medical Jurisprudence*. 13th ed. New York: Churchill Livingstone, 1984.

Thacher, James. *The American New Dispensatory*. Boston: Thomas B. Wait, 1813.

Thomas, Robert. *The Modern Practice of Physic, Exhibiting the Characters, Causes, Symptoms, Prognostic, Marked Appearances, and Improved Method of Treating the Diseases of All Climates*. New York: Collins, 1811.

———. *A Treatise on Domestic Medicine*. New York: Collins, 1822.

Thomas, Theodore G. *A Practical Treatise on the Diseases of Women*. Philadelphia: H. C. Lea, 1868.

Thomson, John. *A Historical Sketch of the Thomsonian System of the Practice of Medicine on Botanical Principles*. Albany: B. D. Packard, 1830.

———. *A Vindication of the Thomsonian System of Practice of Medicine on Botanical Principles*. Albany: Webster and Wood, 1825.

Thomson, Samuel. *New Guide to Health; Or Botanic Family Physician, Containing a Complete System of Practice, Upon a Plan Entirely New: With a Description of the Vegetables Made Use of, and Directions for Preparing and Administering Them to Cure Disease*. 1822. 3d ed. Boston: J. Howe, 1831.

———. *The Thomsonian Materia Medica or Botanic Family Physician: Comprising a Philosophical Theory, the Natural Organization and Assumed Principles of Animal and Vegetable Life: To Which are Added the Description of Plants*. 12th ed. Albany: J. Munsell, 1841.

Thurston, Joseph M. *The Philosophy of Physiomedicalism. Its Theorem, Corollary, and Laws of Application for the Cure of Disease*. Richmond, Ind.: Nicholson Printing and Manufacturing, 1900.

———. *The Principia of Medicine: A Universal Working Hypothesis for a Medical Science*. Richmond, Ind.: J. M. Thurston, 1896.

Tidy, Charles M. *Legal Medicine*. 2 vols. Philadelphia: H. C. Lea's Sons, 1882–84.

Tidy, Charles M., and W. Bathurst Woodman. *On Ammonia in the Urine in Health and Disease*. London: n.p., 1872.

Torrey, Norman L. *Voltaire and the English Deists*. New Haven: Yale University Press, 1930.

Tuke, Daniel Hack. *Illustrations of the Influence of the Mind Upon the Body in Health and Disease: Designed to Elucidate the Action of the Imagination*. Philadelphia: Lindsay and Blakiston, 1872.

Turner, Edward. *Elements of Chemistry. Including the Recent Discoveries and Doctrines of the Science*. Philadelphia: Desilver and Thomas, 1835.

United States Government. Surgeon General's Office. *The Medical and Surgical History of the War of the Rebellion (1861–65). Prepared, in Accordance With the Acts of Congress, Under the Direction of Surgeon General Joseph K. Barnes, United States Army*. 3 parts in 6 vols. Washington, D.C.: Government Printing Office, 1870–88.

Vartanian, Aram, ed. *La Mettrie's L'homme machine: A Study in the Origins of an Idea*. Princeton, N.J.: Princeton University Press, 1960.

Veysey, Lawrence R. *The Emergence of the American University*. Chicago: University of Chicago Press, 1965.

Victor, John. *A History of the Council on Medical Education and Hospitals of the AMA, 1904–1959*. Chicago: American Medical Association, 1959.

Virchow, Rudolph. *Cellular Pathology*. London: John Churchill, 1860.

von Niemeyer, Felix. *A Text-Book of Practical Medicine, With Particular Reference to Physiology and Pathological Anatomy*. 2 vols. New York: D. Appleton, 1869.

Warner, John H. *The Therapeutic Perspective: Medical Practice, Knowledge, and Identity in America, 1820–1885*. Cambridge: Harvard University Press, 1986.

Watson, Patricia Ann. *The Angelical Conjunction: The Preacher-Physicians of Colonial New England*. Knoxville: University of Tennessee Press, 1991.

Watson, Sir Thomas. *Lectures on the Principles and Practice of Physic*. 2 vols. Philadelphia: Blanchard and Lea, 1844.

Weaver, George H. *Beginnings of Medical Education in and Near Chicago; The Institutions and the Men*. Chicago: American Medical Association, 1925.

Weisman, August. *The Germ-Plasm: A Theory of Heredity*. New York: Charles Scribner's Sons, 1893.

———. *The Evolution of Theory*. London: E. Arnold, 1904.

Weisse, Faneuil D. *Practical Human Anatomy, a Working Guide for Students of Medicine and a Ready-Reference for Surgeons and Physicians*. New York: W. Wood, 1886.

Wells, John Soelberg. *A Treatise on the Diseases of the Eye*. Philadelphia: Lindsay and Blakiston, 1870.

Wheeler, Leonard R. *Vitalism: Its History and Vitality*. London: H. F. and G. Witherby, 1939.

Whewell, William. *Philosophy of Inductive Sciences*. 2 vols. New York: Johnson Reprint, 1847.

Whitlaw, Charles. *A Treatise on the Causes and Effects of Inflammation, Fever, Cancer, Scrofula, and Nervous Affections; Observations on the Corrections of Linnaeus's Classification of Diseases*. London: Published by the Author, 1831.

———. *Whitlaw's New Medical Discoveries, With a Defence of the Linnaean Doctrine, and a Translation of His Vegetable Materia Medica, Which Now First Appears in English Dress*. London: Published by Author, 1829.

Whorton, James C. *Crusaders for Fitness: the History of American Health Reformers*. Princeton, N.J.: Princeton University Press, 1982.

Wilder, Alexander. *A History of Medicine: A Brief Outline of Medical History from the Earliest Historic Period With an Extended Account of the Various Sects of Physicians and New Schools of Medicine in Later Centuries*. Augusta, Maine: Maine Farmer Publishing, 1904.

Williams, Henry W. *A Practical Guide to the Study of the Diseases of the Eye: Their Medical and Surgical Treatment*. Boston: Ticknor and Fields, 1862.

Williams, Joseph. *Treatise on the Ear; Including Its Anatomy, Physiology, and Pathology*. London: J. Churchill, 1840.

Wilson, George. *A Handbook of Hygiene and Sanitary Science*. Philadelphia: Blakiston, Son, 1886.

Wilson, W. *Practice of Medicine on Thomsonian Principles*. Memphis, Tenn.: W. Wilson, 1855.

Wilson, Sir William James E. *The Dissector; Or, A Practical and Surgical Anatomy*. Philadelphia: Blanchard and Lea, 1851.

———. *Practical and Surgical Anatomy*. Philadelphia: Lea and Blanchard, 1844.

Windle, Sir Bertran C. A. *What is Life? A Study of Vitalism and Neo-Vitalism*. London: Sands, 1908.

Wistar, Caspar. *A System of Anatomy for the Use of Students of Medicine*. 2 vols. Philadelphia: Thomas, Cowperthwait, 1842–43.

Wood, Alphonso. *Class-Book of Botany: Being Outlines of the Structure, Physiology, and Classification of Plants; With a Flora of the United States and Canada*. New York: Barnes, 1877.

Wood, George B. *Introductory Lecture to the Course of Materia Medica in the University of Pennsylvania*. Philadelphia: J. Young, 1845.

———. *A Treatise on the Practice of Medicine*. Philadelphia: Lippincott, Grambo, 1855.

———. *A Treatise on Therapeutics and Pharmacology or Materia Medica*. 2 vols. Philadelphia: J. B. Lippincott, 1856.

Wood, George B., and Franklin Bache. *The Dispensatory of the United States of America*. Philadelphia: Grigg, Elliot, 1833–49.

———. *The Dispensatory of the United States of America*. Philadelphia: Lippincott, 1866.

Worthy, A. N. *A Treatise on the Botanic Theory and Practice of Medicine*. Forsythe, Ga.: C. R. Hareleiter, 1842.

Wyeth, John Allan. *A Textbook on Surgery, General, Operative, and Mechanical*. New York: D. Appleton, 1887.

Yeo, Gerald F. *A Manual of Physiology. A Textbook for Students of Medicine*. Philadelphia: P. Blakiston, Son, 1888.

Index

xv, 39, 40–42, 67, 73–76, 117, 119; feuds
with Thurston, 121; feuds with White,
117–18; founds physio-medical colleges,
42, 67–78, 139–41; on germ theory,
121–22; as Independent Thomsonian, 67;
on licensing, 76; on material medica,
39–40; on national convention, 116–17,
118, 119, 121, 122, 123; as physio-medical
faculty, 60, 143, 144; as physopath, 67; on
principles of physio-medicine, 40, 67, 68;
on quinine, 101; on regular vs. reform
medicine, 67, 68–70, 72; volunteers for
Union Army, 68, 69; wife of, 103
Cook, William Wesley, 120, 122, 123
Corvisart des Marets, Jean N., 4
Coto bark, 97
Courtney, James, 38
Cousin, Victor, 18
Coutanceau, G. B. A., 18
Coxe, J. Thomas, 46, 47, 60, 113, 114
Credentialing. See Licensing
Culpeper, Nicholas, 12
Curtis, Alva, 30–43, 51, 60; breaks with
Thomson, 30, 33, 112; diplomas granted
or sold by, 40, 42, 43, 58, 62, 67, 73–76,
117; edits journal, 33, 37–38; expands
materia medica, 37; feuds with Cook,
xv, 39, 40–42, 67, 73–76, 117, 119; feuds
with White, 117–18; founds physio-
medicalism, xiii, 13, 38, 42, 63; influence
of, 79; on licensing, 33, 34; on medical
education, 30, 33–34, 43, 48, 49, 57–58;
medical schools founded by, xiii, 33, 34,
35–43, 53, 54, 67, 73, 74, 85–86; medical
society founded by, 112, 113–14; as
Thomsonian, xv, 30–31, 33; and vitalism,
91, 94; on women in medicine, 42–43
Cutler, Manasseh, 12, 103

Darwin, Charles, 90, 92–93
Davidson, G. N. 79
Davis, Nathan Smith, 65
Detwiller, Henry,
Diphtheria, 106–7, 121
Diploma: as license, 128, 129; sold, 40, 42,
43, 58, 62, 67, 73–76, 117, 119
Disease theories (causation theories),
botanic, 28, 47, 109, 114–15; Cook on,
121–22; germ, 105–10, 121–22;

homeopathy on, 9; Koch's 105–6; physio-
medicals on, 102, 109, 120, 121; psora
in, 9; regulars on, 7–8; Rush on, 28;
Thurston on, 128; vitalism on, 90, 94
Drake, Daniel, 72
Dressler, Florence, 173 n. 44
Drug manufacture: botanic/physio, 96, 99;
eclectic, 21, 96–97, 147–48; regular, 96,
97–99, 147–48; Thomson's, 14
Dunglison, Robley, 19
Dynamization, 21

Eaton, Amos, 35
The Eclectic and Medical Botanist, 27
Eclectics, 11, 18–22; Beach and, 13, 19, 50,
59; in California, 22, 127; concentrated
medicines of, xv, 20–21, 22, 58, 59–60;
conciliators, 18, 19; Cook and, 67, 113;
drugs manufactured by, 21, 96–97,
147–48; in France, 18–19; in Georgia, 22,
48; homeopathy's affinity with, 21;
journals of, 27, 127; licensing for, 126,
127; move away from Thomsonism, 28;
national association of, 22, 58, 59; in
Ohio, 20, 22, 58, 62; Paris clinical school
influences, 20; physio-medicals depend
on/turn to, 48, 49–50, 55, 58, 59, 60,
62–63, 95, 96–97, 113, 127, 130, 131,
147–48; physio-medicalism tainted by,
113, 123–24; as reform medicine, 19, 20;
as regular, 113; schools of, 19–20, 21–22,
48, 49–50, 58, 59, 60, 62, 73, 74, 147; on
specific medication, 21, 95; in Tennessee,
49–50
Eclectic Medical College of the City of New
York, 22
Eclectic Medical Institute, 20, 22, 58, 62
Eclectic Medical Institute of Memphis,
49–50
Education, medical, 7–22; admission
requirements in, 3, 5, 6, 57, 62, 81–82,
145, 146; AMA on, 5–6, 65–66, 83–84,
86, 133, 137–38, 139; via apprenticeship,
1, 3; bifurcated, 4; for botanics, 26, 29, 30,
33–34, 35, 43, 45–63, 68, 69, 113, 139;
Civil War affects, 97; clinical access in, 4,
5, 55, 72–73, 81, 82, 84–85, 135–36, 143,
145, 146; curriculum upgraded in, 65–66,
81, 82, 144; eclectic, 19–20, 21–22, 48,

8; hospitals of, 10; journals of, 10; licensing for, 126, 127; "like cures like" theory of, 8–9; materia medica of, 9, 10, 21; medical schools of, 9, 10, 11, 23, 73; numbers of, 11; physios pass as, 130, 131; as reform medicine, 10; regulars convert to, 10; on specific medications, 95; texts of, 10, 23

Hosack, David, 10

Hospitals: access to (*see* Clinical access/studies); homeopathic, 10; physio-medical, 84–85

Howard, Horton, 27–28, 45, 101

Huxley, Thomas Henry, 92

Hydrastis canadensis, 101

Hydro-eclectics, 54

Hydropathy, 55, 56

Illinois: licensing in, 73–74, 76, 122; medical reform in, 133; medical schools in, 10, 65, 73–74, 139, 143, 145, 146, 147 (*see also* Chicago Physio-Medical Institute)

Illinois Medical Practic Act, 73

Illinois State Board of Health: licensing power of, 73–74, 76; on medical schools, 74, 139, 143, 145, 147; reform by, 133

Independent Thomsonian Botanic Society, 30, 112, 113. *See also* Reformed Medical Association of the United States

Independent Thomsonians, xv, 36; on botanic medicines, 112–13; on grangrene, 115; as medical reform, 36–37; medical schools for, 30, 33, 35; national convention of, 111–16. *See also* Curtis, Alva; Cook, William H.; Physio-medicals

Indiana, 129; medical education in, 78–85, 91–94, 130, 145; physio-medicals in, 84–85, 92, 117, 118, 119, 122, 125, 145

Indiana State Sanitarium, 84–85

Indiana University School of Medicine, 85

Jackson, Edward, 23

Jackson, J., 26

James, Samuel, 138

Jenner, Edward, 106

Johns Hopkins Medical School, 136–37

Johnson, H. F., 39, 54, 114

Jones, Ichabod G., 19

Journal of Medical Reform, 47

Journals, 5, 51; botanic, 47, 60 (see also *Worcester Journal of Medicine*); eclectic, 27, 127; homeopathic, 10; reform or physio-medical, 38, 47, 60, 68, 78, 93–94, 97, 109, 119, 124, 126, 130, 131; Thomsonian, 33, 37–38

Keith, Melville C., 99, 103, 119; on diphtheria, 121; on physio-medical convention, 122; on vitalism, 90–91

King, John, 19, 49; on concentrated medicines, 59–60; on eclectic materia medica, 20–21

Koch, Robert, germ theory of, 105–6, 109

Kost, John, 53–54

Laennec, René-Théophile-Hyacinthe, 18

Lavoisier, Antoine Laurent, 91

Lay healers, 12

Licensing, 5, 117, 118, 126–29; AMA on, 137–38; in California, 127; composite boards for, 10, 76, 126, 128–29; Curtis on, 33, 34; diploma as, 128, 129; for eclectics, 126, 127; germ theory and, 108; for homeopaths, 126, 127; in Illinois, 73–74, 76, 122; for physio-medicals, 126, 127; physio-medicals on, 127–28; power of, 3, 66; reciprocal, 129, 131; regulars control, 126–27; repeal of, 111; in Washington, 128

Eli Lilly and Company, 97–99

Lincecum, Gordon, 37

Lincoln Medical College, 22

Lind University, 65

Lippia Mexicana, 97

Literary and Botanico-Medical Institute of Ohio, 35, 45–46. *See also* Botanico-Medical College

Little, Harvey D., 27

Lloyd, John Uri, 21

Lloyd Brothers, Pharmacists, Inc., 97

Lobel, Mathias de, 103

Lobelia: Thomson on, 14, 16, 103–4, 105; uses of, 95, 103–5, 107

Louis, Pierre Charles Alexandre, 19

Loyola University School of Medicine, 147

Ludmerer, Kenneth M., 6

Kindly Medicine

was designed by Will Underwood;

composed in 10½/13 Linotype Goudy Old Style

on a Macintosh Quadra system in QuarkXPress

by The Book Page, Inc.;

printed by sheet-fed offset lithography on

50-pound Lions Falls Turin Book Natural Vellum stock

(an acid-free, totally chlorine-free paper),

notch bound over 88-point binder's boards

in Arrestox B cloth with Multicolor endpapers,

and wrapped with dust jackets printed in three colors

on 100-pound enamel stock finished with

polypropylene film lamination

by Thomson-Shore, Inc.;

and published by

The Kent State University Press

KENT, OHIO 44242